The 15 Minute Fix
VISION

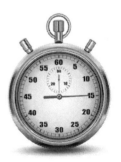

The 15 Minute Fix

Everyday Maintenance For Body, Mind, and Soul

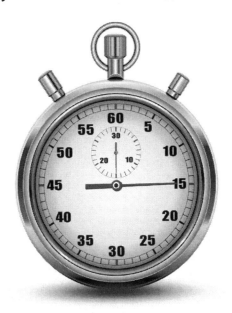

VISION

Eye Exercises Designed To Relieve Stress,
Improve Cognitive Function, Increase Energy
Levels, and Help You See Better

John O. Parker

TIDAL
PUBLISHING

The eye is the jewel of the body.

- Henry David Thoreau

What a curious workmanship is that of the eye, which is in the body, as the sun in the world; set in the head as in a watch-tower, having the softest nerves for receiving the greater multitude of spirits necessary for the act of vision!

- Stephen Charnock

CONTENTS

Welcome to
The 15 Minute Fix

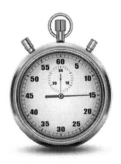

Welcome

Are you having more and more trouble reading books, labels, your phone, or anything else that has small type?

Do you spend the bulk of your day staring at a computer screen?

Have you started to find that vision intensive activities such as driving, computer work, and reading are tiring you out?

If so, <u>The 15 Minute Fix: VISION</u> is here to help. This book will teach you how to use eye exercises to improve or slow the deterioration of your vision, reduce eye strain, and help your brain better interpret the information sent to it by the eyes. You will also learn to use eye exercises to alleviate stress, sharpen cognitive function, increase energy levels, and generally improve your quality of life. If you commit to this program, you will feel like you have a younger pair of eyes, and your overall health will improve.

This book is primarily comprised of a series of eye exercises designed to tone and stretch eye muscles, improve circulation in and around the eyes, train your brain to better understand the signals sent to it by the eyes, and give your eyes a break from their daily work. In addition to the exercises you will find:

- An in depth description of the larger benefits of engaging in eye exercises,

- Tips on how to make your eye exercise program

successful,

- Guidelines on how to develop a workout suited to your particular goals and time/lifestyle constraints,

- Sample workouts to get you started and to generate ideas for creating your own workouts,

- Templates for designing and tracking your workouts,

- Tests to help you track long term changes to your eyes,

- Advice on how to take care of your eyes,

- Information on nutrients that are good for your eyes,

- Suggestions on personal care product ingredients that you should seek out or avoid, and

- A list of resources for learning more about maintaining healthy eyes and vision.

All of this in one handy little book!

Why did I undertake The 15 Minute Fix series?

I pride myself on keeping fit and healthy. I'm not an elite athlete, but I do exercise frequently. I also love preparing for and competing in races – a 5K with the kids, an obstacle course in the mud, an ironman that demands months of preparation, a 24 hour relay race with friends – they're all great. However, even without the races, I would still train. I know that if I don't, I will put on weight, sleep poorly, have less energy, and probably be plain old grumpy. I also find that as I get older, things start to fall apart very quickly if I'm not keeping fit. If I have to take time off for an injury, it takes forever to get my whole body back into shape, not just the injured part. So I do my best to keep fit and healthy. As a result, I feel pretty youthful.

However, as I settled into my 40's, I realized that my usual running, swimming, biking, and gym work kept only a portion of my body healthy. Granted, it is a significant portion (muscles, heart, lungs, etc.), but there are other parts of my body that are also important, and I was doing nothing to keep them in shape. I had never purposefully exercised anything from my neck up (brain, eyes, ears, nose, mouth, face, and scalp). I hadn't focused on taking specific steps to maintain good balance, posture, or motor skills as I "matured." Nor had I developed specific regimes to exercise parts of my body prone to injury (except when I actually had an injury).

Since I have a basic desire to stay active and healthy for as long as possible, I decided to see if there was anything I should be doing to get myself in better overall shape.

First I did some research. I talked to and read papers by established medical experts, alternative health practitioners, and people who will try anything. Many of the exercises and techniques that came out of this research are proven to be beneficial. Others are more controversial but have good potential and general health benefits that make them worth including.

I knew from the outset that some of the approaches I researched were a little on the crazy side. However, as I researched the potential of the intended benefit of a particular exercise or technique, I often found that there were side benefits that made it worth doing even if there was insufficient scientific evidence to prove that it would help achieve its primary purpose. For example, there is little concrete medical data to support the view that scalp exercises will lead to new hair growth. However, there is good anecdotal evidence indicating that scalp exercises will help some people grow new hair and help others keep the hair they've got. What really got me excited, though, were the potential benefits of improving circulation, nerve sensation, and muscle control in all parts of the head. These benefits include stress relief, improved cognitive function, and increased energy levels. All of these are more important to me than my hair (although there is nothing wrong with a full head of hair).

Other areas of interest appeared to require straightforward physical exercise programs on the surface, but devolved into a world of crazy ideas and theories as I dug in further. A great example of this is the Achilles tendon. The Achilles tends to get tighter and tighter as we age, and active people frequently battle Achilles tendonitis. On the surface, there are a number of straightforward exercises to help keep the Achilles stretched and loose. Dig down a bit and talk to people who have tried to manage or recover from Achilles tendonitis, and you find an incredibly stubborn problem that plagues people for months and years. The remedies people try in their quests to fix their Achilles easily rival anything going on in the hair loss world. These include salves, supplements, tape, magnets, splints, boots, massage, scraping, acupuncture, wraps, lifts, orthotics, ultrasound, injections, drugs, and surgery. It's not to say that these remedies can't work, but few of them work for everyone, and some have risks or costs that are unacceptable to many. Trying to find your way through this maze of information is no easy task.

Once I had researched a variety of subjects, I began to experiment based on what I had learned. I practiced the exercises myself to find out which approaches had the best potential and could be done by normal, busy people. Some exercises needed modification, and others needed to be removed because they didn't pass the "normal person" test. Finally, I built a series of exercise programs around this research and called it The 15 Minute Fix.

Fix? Huh?

You may have something you think is broken that you would like to fix, and I encourage you to use these exercises to do just that. However, that's not The 15 Minute Fix. I'd rather you use the exercises as a preventative measure – hopefully making it so that you don't need to be fixed.

So, what do I actually mean by "fix?" OK, don't flip out on me, but I want you to develop an addiction. The best way to get the most out of these exercises is to do them habitually every day. I want you to feel like you need your exercise "fix" every day. You don't need to commit a lot of time, but you do need to commit a little time on a regular basis.

At the outset, this will be difficult. You'll forget to do the exercises. You'll put them off until you have more time. You'll lose your tracking sheet. There is always something (at least there is for me). Each book in the series gives tips on how to design workouts that fit into your lifestyle, but at the end of the day you will simply have to work hard to make your exercise program habitual. Once it is though, your exercises and your progress will happen automatically.

15 minutes? Really?

Yes! On average, 15 minutes a day should do it. However, the objective here is not simply to give each workout a time limit, but rather to help you design a program that is short enough that you have no excuse for not doing it every day. If you want to focus on balance, for example, 15 minutes of balance exercises each day should noticeably improve your balance within a few weeks. After some period of time, perhaps weeks, perhaps months, your exercises will have become a habit, and your focus will shift away from improving your balance to maintaining it. At this point you may find that you can scale back the amount of time you need to put into these particular exercises (although you may find that they are so ingrained in your routine, that it's hard to scale back). Freeing up some time can be particularly helpful if you want to add a new 15 Minute Fix program to your routine.

If you want to tackle 2-4 different 15 Minute Fix programs at once – which I recommend – you will need to budget more than 15 minutes a day. But if you structure your workouts carefully, and they become habitual, you won't feel like you've spent much time doing the workouts. When you take a break at work, you can do an eye exercise, a memory exercise and a balance exercise in five or six minutes. Do that five times a day and you have spent half an hour, without really cutting into your day.

Most of the exercises can be done almost anywhere without specialized equipment. Many can be done while waiting in the airport, on the sidelines of the kids' soccer game, or during a work break. If you want to spread your exercises out over five three-minute sessions during the course of the day – no problem. If you're trying to get more out of the exercises, add a focused 15 minute session to your five three-minute sessions or add a longer session on the weekend. Occasionally you will find an exercise that benefits more than one of your target areas. Use those to save time. You may also find some exercises that you can do at the same time as another exercise. If that works for you, do it.

The key is to design a routine that you can do most days given your individual constraints. Plan your workouts based on your lifestyle and schedule, but don't be afraid to experiment too. Exercising, whether you're focused on your biceps, your hearing, your posture, or anything else, is a dynamic process. You should be playing with your routine all the time.

You may be wondering why I'm asking you to design your own workouts instead of simply giving you a plan to follow. I am a firm believer in the idea that the best workout is the one you are going to do. There is no "one size fits all" here. You need to design and re-design workouts that target the things you want to work on, that fit your schedule, and that you enjoy.

Will you get thin? Will you get ripped? Will you look younger? Will your hair grow back? Can you throw away your glasses? Will all of your aches and pains go away forever?

Possibly, but you have to be realistic. The first thing to understand about The 15 Minute Fix or any other exercise plan is that your results will be a reflection of the work you put into achieving those results. This does not necessarily mean that you will get better results just by spending more time doing the exercises. The best results will come from identifying your goals, then putting together a plan that is consistent with those goals, fits your schedule, evolves as you progress, and is sustainable over a long period of time. Quality vs. quantity. Discipline vs. "whenever I get around to it." Commitment vs. shortcuts.

The second thing to understand is that your goals and expectations need to be reasonable given your current condition, age, and genetic background. If you are 60 years old and 40 pounds overweight, 15 minutes a day of core exercises on an occasional basis will not give you six-pack abs that will be the envy of the 20 year olds on the beach.

However, 15 minutes of focused work every day along with a common sense approach to lifestyle and eating will help you drop some weight, have more energy, and feel better about yourself. If you stick with it, you can eventually reach your ideal weight, and your abs may at least impress other sexagenarians. More importantly though, you'll live longer and your quality of life will be much better than it otherwise would have been. I am not trying to make you younger – that's outside my power. I'm trying to help you age well.

What do I mean by aging well?

Accept that you will get older, but take steps to keep your

body and brain healthy and vibrant. Stay youthful!

If your goal in picking up this book is simply to avoid wearing glasses because they make you look old, I urge you to set the bar higher. Use this and the other books in The 15 Minute Fix series to transform your daily routine into a lifelong program of keeping your mind and body functioning at their highest possible levels. If you do this, you will find that you look and act more youthful and that you have improved your overall health.

In addition to the main focus area of each book (vision in this case), the exercises in each book in The 15 Minute Fix series will help you age well by:

- Lowering your stress levels,

- Elevating your cognitive function,

- Increasing your energy levels,

- Raising your social confidence,

- Improving your performance at work, and

- Maintaining an active, healthy lifestyle much longer than you otherwise would have.

As you dig into each of The 15 Minute Fix books, you will see that they consist of more than just a group of exercises. Each book will contribute toward a comprehensive lifelong plan to age well.

Does this sound like it requires too much work, discipline, or commitment?

It doesn't. The 15 Minute Fix requires all three of these things, but you can handle it. It's like brushing your teeth. If you never brushed your teeth, you would face a future with rotting (and ultimately no) teeth, a shorter life expectancy because of the relationship between dental health and overall health, and low social confidence because your breath would stink and your smile would be something you kept hidden. If someone then told you that you could easily give yourself a 90% chance of keeping most of your teeth for your whole life, improving your overall health for the rest of your life and even extending your life span, and looking and feeling better about yourself every day, but that you would need to take 3-5 minutes 2-3 times day every day of your life to scrub your teeth clean, would you be willing to take that on? Of course you would. It would be hard at first, and you would need some discipline and commitment to get in the habit of doing it, but before too long the process would become automatic. Just as it will with any 15 Minute Fix program you commit to.

Because it's tough though, you'll find resources to help you at www.the15minutefix.com. There you will find articles, support, and tools to help you find your way.

So, join me as we embark on a lifelong journey of aging well!

Introduction
VISION

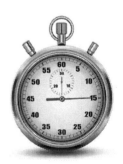

Introduction

When I was three years old, I started to wear glasses. I couldn't stand them. I mean, I just hated them. Luckily, when I was 13, my eye doctor informed me that I no longer needed to wear corrective eyewear. Woo hoo! Let the good times roll! Really, I was thrilled. Since then, however, I have come to understand more about what was going on with my eyes back then.

Basically, the reason for my wearing glasses never really went away. I have amblyopia – basically, I only use one eye. When I was young, it was visibly noticeable and prevented me from developing binocular vision, an essential part of seeing in three dimensions. As I grew older, my eyes straightened out and I became adept at using perspective as a substitute for my lack of depth perception. Essentially, by the time I was 13, I had two very good eyes that just didn't like to work with each other. I was told that by that age, my brain was hard wired to receive input from my eyes this way. End of story. Since then, however, I have learned that there are people out there who have been able to develop binocular vision later in life. They have done it by exercising their eyes.

More recently, a couple of other things led me to think about eye exercises. The first was the insistence of my eye doctor that sooner or later I would need to start wearing glasses again – for an entirely new reason. Specifically, because I'm getting older. Now, I don't mind getting older (it beats the alternative), but I work hard to not let my body and my brain fall apart in the process. Taking care of my eyes as they age, the same way I take care of my body as it ages is only logical to me.

The other thing that really helped me start thinking about my eyes was my lifestyle. I have basically had my eyes glued to books or computers for 40+ hours a week since I was in high school. I came to understand that this has taken a toll on my eyes the same way that driving a cab or a truck for decades has on your legs and back. They're being used, but they are not getting stretched or worked. Nor do they get sufficient oxygen and nutrients. If the legs aren't being taken care of, other things will start to break down because of poor circulation, misaligned hips, etc. Just like my legs would need exercise in this case, I decided that my eyes would benefit from exercise too.

These realizations finally gelled into a wake up call. I decided to start learning about and experimenting with eye exercises. Using the exercises in this book, I have made some remarkable changes in the way I see, think, and feel. I still don't have binocular vision, but the exercises have helped me see better, read for longer periods of time with greater comprehension, and feel more alert and energetic.

Why do eye exercises?

Eye exercises are a wonderful way to relieve stress, improve cognitive function, increase energy levels, and generally improve your quality of life. They can also help athletes at all levels improve their reaction time and orientation to targets.

They may also improve your vision.

Wait... did you say: "May improve your vision?" Isn't improving my vision the whole point of doing these exercises in the first place?

Perhaps, but you need to understand that there are a wide

variety of conditions that can affect your eyes. Many experts claim that many of these conditions cannot be cured. For example, most eye doctors contend that nothing can be done about nearsightedness because it is caused by the shape of your eyeball, which you can't change through exercise. However, there is strong evidence that nearsightedness is largely caused by our environment. Statistics indicate that 100 years ago, around 5% of the U.S. population suffered from myopia (nearsightedness), while today nearly a third of the U.S. population is nearsighted. It stands to reason that the ability to read well into the night, the shift from outdoor jobs to factory jobs to desk jobs, and the introduction of computers are likely reasons for the degeneration of modern eyeballs. Therefore, it stands to reason, that if our environment is causing the damage, then we can take steps to stop or even repair the damage. Just keep in mind, that from a scientific perspective, this is unproven.

There is, however, anecdotal evidence that individuals with a wide range of eye conditions can improve their vision through exercise. If you are suffering from age related eye degeneration (presbyopia), have one eye that is not aligned with the other (strabismus, amblyopia, etc.), suffer from eye strain (eyes that tire easily, headaches from reading or doing computer work, blurry or double vision, sensitivity to bright light, etc.), or simply find that your attention span is decreasing, then eye exercises may help.

In many cases, eye exercises do not technically improve one's vision, rather they train the brain to better process the information it receives through the eyes. Personally, I don't care if it's my brain or my eyes that help me see better – I'm just happy if I can.

So, if the exercises might or might not improve your vision (or if you're perfectly content with your vision), should you bother with eye exercises?

Absolutely! In a day and age when people are glued to their chairs, staring at computer screens for hours and hours all day long, eye exercises are an important part of keeping your eyes and your brain healthy as well as supporting your overall health. In addition to potentially improving your vision, the exercises described in this book are designed to:

- Alleviate and stave off eye strain,

- Relieve stress,

- Raise your mental energy and alertness,

- Help keep you stay awake during long work days,

- Improve reaction time and orientation in sports and other physical activities,

- Allow you to maintain your current vision longer than you otherwise would have, and

- In some cases, improve your vision.

My hope is that you will use these exercises to age well. I want you to have youthful eyes. This may include vision improvement, but if it doesn't, don't sweat it. There are plenty of young and youthful people with imperfect vision, yet they still have eyes that communicate confidence, happiness, desire, wonder, and dozens of other youthful emotions. Exercising your eyes will improve your overall health and give your eyes the means to express your newfound youthfulness.

How do I go about exercising my eyes?

While there are some immediate benefits to doing eye exercises, especially when it comes to relieving stress and boosting energy, long lasting benefits require a plan and commitment. The following guidelines will help make this possible.

Make it a habit: The 15 Minute Fix is all about making a group of targeted exercises part of your daily routine without taking a lot of time or disrupting your life. It's better to do a few exercises each day with intent and focus than to do a bunch of them mechanically once or twice a week. Ultimately, you want to do your exercises habitually, the way you might have a cup of coffee in the morning or brush your teeth after meals. Your goal is to get to the point where you can't live without doing your 5-10 eye exercises a day.

In order to do this though, you need planning, discipline, and commitment. Planning means that you need to think about where and when you will be doing your exercises. Some exercises require you to go someplace or have a little privacy, so don't use these if your plan is to work in exercises over the course of the day at work. Save them for when you have some private time in your schedule.

Discipline means that you need a system in place to make sure you do your exercises. If you are trying to fit your routine into a workday filled with tasks, meetings, phone calls, distractions, and exhaustion, you will need help remembering to do your exercises. You might want to set a timer to remind you to give your eyes a break and do one or two exercises every hour (particularly if you're trying to relieve eye strain). If your timer goes off at an inconvenient time, taking even a tiny break of 30-60 seconds to do some kind of eye movement is beneficial.

If a timer doesn't work for you, tie your exercises to moments of down time that repeat. For example, when your computer takes its sweet time to do something (PCs and Macs both use a "busy" timer that can be a great visual clue), do a particular exercise or just make a few circles with your eyes. Do this every time your computer is busy and you should notice that your eyes aren't as tired as usual at the end of the day. Do it enough, and it will become automatic.

If you spend a lot of time on the phone, keep a tracking sheet next to your phone to remind you to do some exercises while you're on hold or listening to a conference call. If you travel, make it part of your routine to do some manageable (i.e. not too embarrassing) exercises every time you ride in a taxi, sit on a train, or wait at a departure gate. I see no reason why you shouldn't fit in an exercise or two while you're in the bathroom (multi-tasking is a valuable skill these days). Find those unproductive moments in your day and take advantage of them with a planned routine. If you do it with enough frequency and consistency, you will find yourself doing the exercises without even thinking about it. That's when you know you're on the right track!

Make a long term commitment: If you intend to be one of the subset of people who actually improve their vision, you will need dedication and perseverance. You do not need to spend a huge amount of time on any given day – 15 minutes should do it – but you will need to practice at least three days a week and preferably six days a week for an extended period of time. We're not talking days and weeks here. We're talking about months and years. You are embarking on a program to keep your eyes healthy for the rest of your life.

Keep expectations reasonable: As with any exercise program, it is important to not expect the impossible when undertaking an eye exercise program. With eyes in particular, I urge you to use the exercises for stress relief, improving mental focus, general health benefits and maintaining your current vision. If your vision improves, consider it a bonus.

I would also suggest that when it comes to your eyes, you not let vanity get the better of your common sense - if you need glasses, wear them. Take them off while performing most of the eye exercises, but only to the extent that you can do the exercise with out putting undue strain on your eyes. Then put your glasses back on as you go about your daily activities. If your prescription needs change, your eye doctor will let you know.

Track your progress: Tracking eye workouts is different than tracking a typical gym workout. There are no weights to record and reps are often meaningless. Nevertheless, it is still helpful to track what exercises you are doing, how your eyes feel before and after, and how long you practice your exercises. Recording the details of your exercises will allow you to pinpoint which exercises are most effective for you, which ones may be losing their impact, and how time of day, amount of time spent practicing your exercises, and your general mood affect the benefit you get. If you can remember to note how your eyes feel a couple of hours later, that too will provide you with an important data point.

In addition to everyday exercise tracking, it is helpful to test your vision on a regular basis. This will allow you to track actual changes over time. Appendix 1 has a series of self-administered vision tests that will give you a baseline and consistent means for tracking any improvement.

Stay focused but relaxed: When you're doing eye exercises, it is helpful to be in the right frame of mind. You are not engaging in weightlifting for the eyes, so you do not need a Red Bull and protein shake before you start. Your eyes are working all of the time - you do not need to build muscle around your eyes. Rather, you want to improve muscle flexibility and range of motion, like yoga for the eyes. Before you begin your routine do the warm-up exercise (#1) or other *Relaxation* exercises. If you are only taking time to do one or two exercises, take several deep breaths with your eyes closed before you start. Once engaged in your workout, do your exercises intently and diligently – no punching the clock here.

The trick is to differentiate between physical exertion (bad) and mental concentration (good). This will help you achieve a balance between relaxation and focus.

Also, if you find, at any time, that your eye exercise routine is giving you a headache, making you squint, or otherwise not leaving you more rested and alert than when you started - scale back until you find a routine that leaves you in better shape than when you started. If you wear contacts, be aware that occasionally they can suction to the eyeball or move around while doing eye exercises. If this happens regularly, figure out which exercises you can do without having problems and save the rest for when you have your contacts out.

Cross-train: Eye strain and its symptoms often come from focusing on one thing at a fixed distance for too long. These days, that usually means spending too long staring at a computer screen, but there are many other activities that can cause you to look in one place for hours. Human eyes are not designed for books or computer screens. They evolved to help us see at a variety of distances, while moving at different speeds, and in natural light. Think about what happens to the muscles in your arm or leg if they are in a cast for a few weeks. They atrophy. If you spend day after day simply staring at your computer, a similar thing can happen to your eyes.

By forcing you to use your eyes in a variety of new and different ways, eye exercises inherently cross train your eyes. Additionally, however, I would urge you to mix a wide variety of exercises into your weekly routine. If you will be focusing your efforts on a specific vision concern, be sure to include a couple of exercises that are general in nature or target other concerns. And rather than put together one plan you use every day, keep you eyes from getting used to a routine by making a weekly plan that mixes up the daily routine. Instead of doing the same 5-10 exercises every day, try to do 15-20 different exercises over the course of the week. If there are one or two exercises that that really make your eyes feel better or give your brain a serious kick start, by all means, use them frequently, but shuffle your other exercises around. If you find yourself just punching the clock with an exercise, cycle it out of your routine for a bit. Mixing up your routine, will keep your eyes and brain engaged.

How do I figure out which eye exercises I should do?

At the outset, you may want to start with one or two of the sample plans in Appendix 2. Once you settle in however, I encourage you to develop your own routine, incorporating exercises that have given you positive results (once you have been doing them long enough to have sufficient data), that make you feel good, that you enjoy, and that fit your schedule. Remember, If your plan doesn't fit your schedule or is unpleasant to do, it won't work.

The exercises in this book fall into the following general categories:

1. *Relaxation exercises*

These exercises relieve eye strain, improve your energy levels, and keep your brain sharp. By forcing you to relax while stimulating blood flow, which brings oxygen and nutrients to your eyes, these exercises can be used to rest your eyes and energize them at the same time. Use these exercises to give yourself a quick break and to warm up and cool down at the beginning and end of your routine. These exercises are an important part of maintaining your overall health.

2. *Flexibility exercises*

These exercises train your eyes to move and focus (accommodate), thereby improving flexibility, range of motion, and focal variability. They are particularly helpful in managing eye conditions that respond to therapy, including early presbyopia.

In addition to improving your ability to move and focus your eyes, these exercises will train your eye muscles and your brain to work together in a more effective manner. We all inevitably develop bad eye habits. You will benefit from practicing exercises that enforce good eye habits. Just as a baseball player or a golfer needs to take thousands upon thousands of swings to ingrain the right movements into their "muscle memory", you need to practice all of the ways you might use your eyes in order for them to "remember" how to function to the best of their ability.

When practicing flexibility exercises, remember to keep your eyes relaxed and not push them too far. It is possible to strain your eyes doing exercises, so relax, breathe, and don't overdo it in any one session. Of course, the best way to manage this is to work a series of stress reduction exercises into any training routine.

3.   *Targeted exercises*

These exercises are designed to help you improve one or more of the following:

- Near vision
- Distance vision
- Binocular vision and depth perception
- Peripheral vision
- Tracking and sports training

Of course, many exercises fit into more than one category, and all of them will help keep your eyes limber and stimulate the vision center of the brain, so don't be afraid to practice any of the exercises, even if one type suits your objectives better. That having been said, these categorizations should help you figure out which exercises you want to add to your routine.

I suggest that you build your eye exercise routine in three stages:

1. One or two warm-up and circulation exercises,

2. A core group of exercises targeted toward areas of particular concern , and

3. A couple of general exercises including at least one *Relaxation* exercise and one *Flexibility* exercise.

Again, Appendix 2 has some templates you can use to get started, but don't be afraid to experiment. Play around with different exercises, even those that do not seem to target your main goals. Track how each exercise feels, how much time it takes, how it fits with your lifestyle, etc. Within a few weeks you will have a good feel for what works for you.

Over time, remember to strike a balance between giving an exercise time to work and bringing new exercises into your routine. If you have been doing the same routine for a couple of months, make sure to add some new exercises to your routine for a bit, even if you have to swap out a favorite for a period of time.

Is there anything else I can do to keep my eyes healthy?

Take care of yourself: Eat well (lots of lean protein and vegetables and as little processed food as possible), drink plenty of water (4-6 big glasses a day), get enough sleep (7+ hours if possible), breathe deeply throughout the day, and exercise or at least make sure you get up and move around on a regular basis. If you smoke, please stop. Doing these things will help your immune system, your circulation, and your cognitive function, all of which will help you maintain healthy eyes. (Appendix 5 discusses foods which may be extra beneficial to the eyes.)

If you are tired or sick or if your eyes are worn out from an earlier round of eye exercises, take a day off from any strenuous exercises. Focus on exercises that will relax your eyes on those days.

Feed your eyes with light: Go outdoors in the sunlight every day. Even cloudy days provide a tremendous amount of sunlight. The best time to get sunlight is in the morning and the evening, when the sun is somewhat lower in the sky (remember to never look directly at the sun). Avoid overusing sunglasses as they prevent healthy adjustments of the iris that keep your eyes in shape. Try to limit your use of sunglasses to when it is necessary (e.g. driving into a sunrise or sunset).

When you are inside, make sure you have sufficient light when you are using your eyes (reading, working, cooking, etc.) Low light causes unnecessary eye strain.

Protect your eyes: When you do use sunglasses make sure they offer adequate protection. When purchasing sunglasses, look for ones that block out 99 to 100 percent of both UV-A and UV-B radiation. If you have dry eyes, keep your eyes hydrated through preservative-free artificial tears and/or the use of clean humidifiers. Wear protective eyewear while doing work or leisure activities that can damage the eyes (using power tools or chemicals, playing sports, etc.)

Wear your seatbelt: A common cause of problems with all senses is automobile accidents, even low-speed crashes. Beside the risk of direct damage to your eyes, a strong impact can shift the brain within your skull, tearing delicate nerve fibers that connect your eyes and everything else in your body to your brain.

Wait, let's get back to eye exercises, what's it going to take to improve my vision?

Dedication and perseverance. If you want to improve your eyesight (and as I discussed at the beginning, there are no guarantees), you must make eye exercises a long term habit. You don't need to spend more than 15 minutes a day, but you should exercise frequently (preferably 5-6 days a week) with focus and intent. Track your progress for 12 months. You'll know by that point whether or not your efforts are resulting in improved vision.

Remember, it's not just about improving your vision. A year of consistently following an eye exercise plan will help alleviate stress, increase your mental sharpness, boost your energy levels, and help you feel healthier and more youthful.

Healthy, youthful eyes are within reach! Let's get to work!

How to use
this book

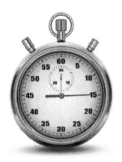

How to use this book

The exercises in this book are meant to be self-explanatory, but just in case, here is a guide to the layout and symbols found on the following pages.

The Exercise

Each exercise and test is numbered (on its Difficulty Rating) and has a unique title. The main body of each page explains how to set up for each exercise and how to execute it.

Difficulty Rating

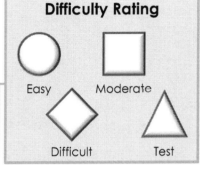

Easy   Moderate

Difficult   Test

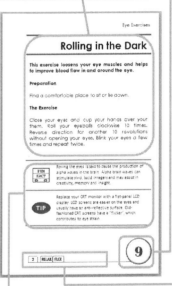

Benefits & Uses

RELAX	Relaxation/Stress Relief
FLEX	Flexibility
NEAR	Near Vision
FAR	Distance Vision
3D	Binocular Vision/Depth
SIDE	Peripheral Vision
TRACK	Tracking/Sports Training
3	Expected Minutes

Extras

Suggestions for taking an exercise to the next level or to add an optional component.

Useful tips relating to both specific exercises and general care of your vision.

Interesting tidbits that don't require or even suggest you do anything else.

Tips
Get the most out of your eye exercise routine

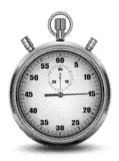

These tips will help you get the most out of your eye exercise routine.

- Wash your hands before doing eye exercises (or whenever you touch around your eyes) to avoid getting irritants in your eyes and to prevent the spread of disease.

- Close your eyes and take several long, deep breaths before you begin.

- Except where instructed to cover your eyes, do your exercises in good light, preferably bright, indirect sunlight.

- Unless otherwise instructed, keep eye movements smooth and relaxed.

- Do not apply heavy pressure to your eyes.

- Do not directly touch your eyes.

- If your eyes tend to become dry, get some preservative free artificial tear eye drops and use them before you do your exercises (or other times during the day when your eyes feel tired or dry.)

- If your eyes feel sore or fatigued from exercising them, ease up or take a break for a couple of days to let them rest and recover.

- Stay hydrated, give your body the proper nutrients it needs, and get enough sleep.

- Do <u>not</u> do eye exercises while driving.

- Do <u>not</u> do eye exercises in the middle of a date or in front of criminal-types who do not like to be looked at funny.

The Exercises

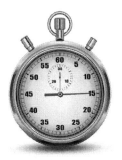

5x5 Warm-Up

Use this as a warm up before performing other eye exercises or on its own to increase the blood flow to your eyes and relieve eyestrain.

Preparation

Sit in a quiet room and close your eyes.

The Exercise

1. Take five full, deep breaths.

2. Breathing in, nod your head slowly up and exhale down five times.

3. Keeping your spine straight and your neck relaxed, breathe your head to the right as far as it will comfortably go, exhale back to center, and repeat on the left. Do this five times on both sides.

4. Breathing steadily, drop your head forward and roll it in a wide circle five times in both directions.

5. Roll your right shoulder up and forward then back and down. Do the same with the left shoulder before rolling both shoulders at once. Again – five times.

1

20-20-20

Use this quick exercise to reduce eye fatigue if you spend a lot of time reading, working at the computer, or focusing on close-up details.

Preparation

Do this exercise after every 20-30 minutes of close-up focusing.

The Exercise

Look at an object that is about 20 feet away. With relaxed eyes, focus on the object for 20 seconds then return to your work.

 Stand up and do 10 air squats after each set to improve overall body health.

 Use a timer to remind you to take your break. 20 minutes can fly by!

| RELAX | FAR | ½ |

Palming

An effective way to reset your eyes and mind when they become tired and lose focus.

Preparation

Sit comfortably on a chair with your elbows resting on a desk, table, or your knees. Clear your mind and breathe deeply.

The Exercise

With closed eyes, rub your palms together until they feel warm. Breathing deeply, place your palms over your eyes without touching your eyelids or covering your nose. Let the heels of your hands rest on your cheekbones and let your fingers overlap on your forehead. Try to block all light from coming in. Open your eyes and focus on the darkness. You may see traces of light but focus on the blackness. Hold until you see only blackness or up to three minutes. Repeat whenever your eyes feel strained.

 Try Palming in a fetal kneeling position (kneeling with butt on heels and forehead on the floor) for deeper relaxation.

Sleepy Eyes

A great quick eye relaxation exercise.

Preparation

Sit or lie in a relaxed, comfortable position.

The Exercise

Close your eyes halfway and concentrate on stopping your eyelids from trembling. You will find that this requires you to relax your eyes. Once your eyelids stop trembling, shift your gaze to a far off object while maintaining your relaxed state.

Hold for up to a minute, then repeat 2-3 times.

 Don't squint or hold your eyelids in place with the muscles around your eyebrows. Stay relaxed, moving only the eyelids.

 Blink a few times between sets of this and any exercise with multiple sets.

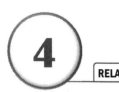

Blinking

An often overlooked yet simple way to keep your eyes fresh and able to focus longer.

Preparation

This can be done pretty much anytime and anywhere.

The Exercise

Spend 15 seconds blinking rapidly, followed by 45 seconds of blinking every 3-4 seconds.

Do this twice.

Humans use blink rate to communicate with others. When someone stops blinking and stares at you while you are talking, it's a sign of aggression. However whenever you are talking to someone and they are blinking at 4-5 second intervals it's a sign of a relaxed and friendly listener.

Computer users and television watchers tend to blink less, especially when they are intently focused on something.

5

Relaxed Eyes

Give your eyes a break after a stressful day by focusing on nothing. This should completely relax tired eyes.

Preparation

Sit or lie somewhere quiet with soft or natural lighting.

The Exercise

Look towards an area with as few objects or defined shapes as possible and relax your eyes so that they are not focused on anything in particular. Avoid focusing on any objects or shapes that remain in your line of sight. Relax your gaze and concentrate your attention on your breathing.

Hold for five minutes.

This exercise can be difficult to master because our eyes are used to being focused. If you are having trouble focusing on nothing, practice the exercise in front of a surface with little spatial context, such as a wall painted in a solid color, lying under a plain white ceiling or looking up at the clear blue sky.

6

RELAX

Phantom Sight

Relax your eyes while developing your brain's ability to interpret what it sees.

Preparation

Lie on your back or sit comfortably looking forward at an object or mark on the ceiling or wall. What you are looking at should have a distinct shape and have a relatively blank backdrop.

The Exercise

Focus on your shape. After 30 seconds, close your eyes for one complete breath (in and out) and continue to "see" (visualize) your object. Open your eyes and refocus on the shape for another complete breath. Repeat the cycle of closing and opening your eyes while visualizing and refocusing on your shape 10 times.

 Don't use a light that is on as your object.

 If your ceiling or wall does not have a distinct shape, tape something to it.

7

Visualization

This exercise helps relax the eyes and improve concentration.

Preparation

Ideally, you want to be lying on your back when doing this one, but sitting comfortably at your desk is fine too.

The Exercise

Close your eyes and breathe deeply for about a minute. Open your eyes and focus on an object for 30 seconds. Close your eyes again and, breathing deeply, visualize the object in your head for another 30 seconds. Repeat opening and closing your eyes two more times.

 If you are lying down, it can be hard to find good objects to visualize. Ceiling fans or unlit light fixtures work well.

 Once you can visualize an object with relative ease, try looking at a different object each time you open your eyes.

8

Rolling In The Dark

This exercise loosens your eye muscles and helps improve blood flow in and around the eye.

Preparation

Find a comfortable place to sit or lie down.

The Exercise

Close your eyes and cup your hands over them. Roll your eyeballs clockwise 10 times. Reverse direction for another 10 revolutions without opening your eyes. Blink your eyes a few times and repeat twice.

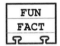

Rolling the eyes is said to cause the production of alpha waves in the brain. Alpha brain waves can stimulate vivid, lucid imagery and may assist in creativity, memory and insight.

Replace your CRT monitor with a flat-panel LCD display. LCD screens are easier on the eyes and usually have an anti-reflective surface. Old-fashioned CRT screens have a "flicker," which contributes to eye strain.

Eye Squeeze

Engages and then relaxes eye muscles to help combat eye stress and strain.

Preparation

Sitting with good posture, relax your shoulders, neck, and head.

The Exercise

Look straight ahead, inhale, and open your eyes and mouth as wide as you can. Exhale deeply, shut your eyes and mouth, and squeeze your eyes and other facial muscles as tight as you can. When you squeeze your eyes shut you should feel the muscles around your eyes contract. Hold the squeeze while exhaling for 5-10 seconds, release quickly, and relax your open eyes for three to four seconds while inhaling.

Repeat this movement up to 10 times.

Eye squeezes increase the flow of blood and oxygen to your entire face, making this an excellent exercise when you need a quick energy boost.

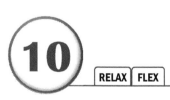

RELAX | FLEX

Rockin'

Practice picking up fine detail at variable close distances.

Preparation

Sit or stand with one foot in front of the other about three feet in front of a Near Eye Chart.

The Exercise

Focus on a letter in the smallest row that you can see clearly. Rock back and forth while maintaining focus on the letter. If necessary, adjust your position so that you are nearing the boundaries of your range of focus (without straining your eyes).

Rock for one minute, blink a few times and repeat.

 Breath in deeply as you rock back and out fully as you rock forward.

Compass Points

This Ayurvedic exercise is especially beneficial to those suffering from dry or red eyes (often a result of working on a computer all day).

Preparation

Sit comfortably.

The Exercise

With your eyes open and head still, look up as far as you can and hold for three seconds. Close the eyes and hold for two seconds. Open the eyes and look all the way down, again holding for three seconds. Close the eyes and hold for two seconds. Repeat the above while looking to the right side and then to the left. Repeat the series five times.

 Be sure not to force your eyes further than they want to go in any particular direction.

 Ayurvedic medicine is a system of traditional healing that originated in ancient India.

Distance Focusing

Give the eyes a rest from up-close work including reading, paperwork, and computer use.

Preparation

Find an outdoor spot where you can see fairly far.

The Exercise

Focus on the farthest object you can see and notice the difference in clarity between that object and something closer. Hold your focus on the distant object for an entire minute.

Repeat two more times with other similarly far objects.

 Bring your hand into focus between sets to reset your eyes.

 Do eye exercises in sunlight whenever possible. Lack of sunlight may be a significant contributor to developing myopia.

Steady Gaze

Weak eyes have trouble focusing on a single spot. Use this exercise to improve your ability to hold your eyes steady.

Preparation

Can be done pretty much anytime you can focus on a still object (i.e. not when you're moving).

The Exercise

Breathe naturally and keep your face relaxed. While focusing on an object (near or far), hold your eyes still for 30 seconds at a time (it's OK to blink). Close your eyes for 10 seconds, then repeat 5-7 times.

As you become proficient, vary your distances and try to hold your eyes still for longer periods of time. Don't be concerned if your eyes start to tear while holding your eyes steady for longer periods of time.

FUN FACT The ability to hold eye contact with a steady gaze shows confidence and (along with a smile) makes a person more attractive.

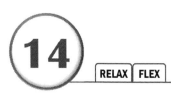

RELAX | FLEX

Near-Far

Will relax tired eyes and may improve vision.

Preparation

Grasp a pencil or other small object (or just use your finger) and hold it at arms length.

The Exercise

Hold the pencil as close to your nose as you can without it blurring and focus on it for 30 seconds. Then, slowly shift your focus to something on the other side of the room (or 10-20 feet away) that you can see in clear focus. Again, hold your focus for 30 seconds. Repeat the sequence. After the first two sets, shift your focus between the objects with each in and out breath. Repeat this quicker near-far shift 5-10 times.

 Try this exercise outside or at a window with the far object at least 100 feet away.

 Move the pencil progressively closer (but still in focus) from session to session.

15

Sunning

A relaxation exercise that also works the iris by bathing it in light.

Preparation

Sit comfortably facing the sun with closed eyes. Relax your neck and shoulders while breathing deeply. This is best done mid-morning or late afternoon.

The Exercise

With eyes closed, gently turn your head back and forth, from shoulder to shoulder, with the sun shining on your eyelids. "Watch" the sun move back and forth at a moderate pace. Continue for 3-5 minutes.

Finish with Palming.

 Be sure not to look directly at the sun during this exercise. Don't squeeze your eyes closed – keep them relaxed but fully closed.

Trataka

This Ayurvedic exercise can be a good exercise for those with depth perception issues.

Preparation

Sit comfortably at arms length in front of a lit candle while breathing naturally.

The Exercise

Gaze steadily at the candle flame, without blinking or moving your body. Continue staring until your eyes start to water. Open your eyes wider and hold until tears drip down your cheeks. Finally, close your eyes and try to visualize the candle flame for as long as possible.

Try to work your way up to five minutes of staring before closing your eyes.

Trataka has been used for eye cleansing and meditation by yogis since ancient times. Similar exercises were practiced by early adherents of Christianity, Islam, and Judaism.

17

Four Corners

Improve your peripheral vision and stretch your eye muscles at the same time.

Preparation

Sit in a room facing the center of a wall at a distance where you can just focus on the corners of the room without turning your head.

The Exercise

Keeping your head still, look up with both eyes toward the upper right corner of the room, and then down to the lower left corner. Repeat the exercise, switching your gaze to the upper left and lower right then blink and rest the eyes. Repeat both movements four times.

Once you are used to this exercise, move your chair two feet closer to the wall in front of you after each rep. This will add a depth component to this range exercise.

Peripheral vision is an important component of your ability to remain balanced.

Big Ben

A simple and effective way to work on developing your peripheral vision.

Preparation

Sit, lie, or stand in a relaxed, comfortable position.

The Exercise

Imagine that you are in front of a ten foot tall clock about five feet away. Look at the middle of the clock (eye level if you are standing). Then look at any hour mark, without turning your head. Look back at the center. Repeat with the other 11 hour marks (in any order). Let your eyes move to the edge of their natural range, but do not strain them.

 Over time, change the imaginary distance of your clock, from session to session. Try seeing a clock both closer and much further.

 You can also do this exercise with your eyes closed.

Figure Eight

A fluid way to develop eye flexibility and peripheral vision.

Preparation

Sit or lie in a relaxed, comfortable position.

The Exercise

Without moving your head, slowly trace an imaginary figure eight lying on its side. Let your eyes move to the edge of their natural range, but do not strain them.

Do this for 1-2 minutes, then reverse direction for the same amount of time.

Try to move your eyes with a "weighted" rhythm, as if gravity were causing your eyes to accelerate on the downslope and decelerate on the up slope. The feeling of this rhythm will increase the meditative effect of the exercise.

Simple Trombone

This exercise can help develop your focusing skills, particularly if you have convergence insufficiency (when your eyes don't turn inward properly while you're focusing on a nearby object).

Preparation

Grasp a pencil or other small object (or just use your finger) and hold it in front of you at arm's length.

The Exercise

Focus on the pencil. Slowly bring the pencil in toward your nose, continuing to focus on the pencil as it moves. Stop before you see two pencils or when it is three inches from your nose. Hold for a moment and then slowly move the pencil away until your arm is fully outstretched again. Repeat for 2-3 minutes.

 TIP When finished, relax with eyes closed for one minute. Do this with all "focusing" exercises.

Single-Eye Trombone

If Simple Trombone is difficult, start by developing greater eye control and flexibility with this exercise.

Preparation

Get an object like a pencil with some clear print on it.

The Exercise

Cover your left eye with your left hand (keeping the eye open). Hold the pencil in front of your right eye with your right hand and, focusing on the print, slowly move it away from you. Move the pencil all the way out and all the way in, even past the point of clear vision. Retain your focus as long as you can in each direction. If you lose focus, complete the directional movement and try to recapture focus as soon as possible after reversing direction.

Do this in and out movement for a minute before repeating with the left eye.

 Finish by trying a couple Simple Trombone reps.

FLEX | NEAR   TRACK | 2

Complex Trombone

A series of "trombone" exercises that is practically a full eye workout by itself.

Preparation

Grasp a pencil or other small object with print on it and hold it in front of you at arm's length.

The Exercise

Cover your left eye with one hand (keeping the eye open). Without moving your head, focus on the print with your right eye. slowly bring the pencil in toward your forehead, stopping before you lose focus. Maintaining focus, slowly extend your arm then bring the pencil toward your chin. Do three sets with each eye and then with both eyes.

Next, repeat the sequence (each eye individually then both eyes) moving the pencil from side to side as far as you can about a foot in front of you.

Next, repeat the sequence moving the pencil from arms length straight in front of you to each shoulder.

Finally, run through the sequence tracing a large (three foot) circle in front of you (going both ways) and a small (one foot) circle in front of you.

Text Trombone

Tromboning for reading improves flexibility in your eye muscles.

Preparation

Sit comfortably holding a Near Eye Chart.

The Exercise

Starting about 12 inches from your face, look at a line of larger text (line 4 or 5 should work well) and move it away from your eyes until you can see it very clearly. Slowly move the text closer, until it begins to blur. Continue to move the text in and out slowly. You will probably notice that you progressively bring the chart closer with each rep. Once you can read the line clearly from six inches away, switch to a smaller line (6, 7, or 8) and repeat the exercise. Do this for a couple of minutes 2-3 times a day. Adjust which lines you use based on your ability to ultimately see the letters clearly when they are six inches from your face.

 Once adept at this exercise, practice reading small print in different kinds of light (but never so dim as to cause eye strain).

FLEX | NEAR | 3D | 5

Pencil Focus

This convergence exercise engages eye muscles while focusing on a small point.

Preparation

Get a pencil or other small object with writing on it. Stand or sit with straight back and shoulders down away from your ears. Relax your shoulders, neck, and head while looking straight ahead.

The Exercise

Hold the pencil at arm's length in front of your nose. Focus both eyes on a letter on the pencil and slowly bring the pencil toward your nose. Hold your gaze on the letter until you lose focus, then extend the pencil back out to arm's length. Repeat this movement 5-10 times.

FUN FACT

Golfers often adjust their head position and posture (to the detriment of their swing) to compensate for strabismus or the dominance of one eye. Convergence exercises like this will help keep the eyes balanced.

Telescoping

Good for improving the eyes' ability to move between near and far focal points.

Preparation

Sit or stand comfortably outside or at a window where you can see for a good distance.

The Exercise

Start by focusing on the tip of your nose. After five seconds, move your finger 12 inches in front of your nose and focus on it. After another five seconds shift your focus to a nearby object (within five feet.) Continue shifting your focus to 10, 20, 50, 100, 200, and if you can, 500 feet away. Focus for five seconds at each of the distances.

Repeat three times.

Hawks have telescopic vision that allows them to spot prey from a mile away. However, this comes at the expense of peripheral vision.

FLEX | NEAR | FAR   TRACK | 2

Distant To Close

This Ayurvedic exercise is excellent for athletes with depth perception issues.

Preparation

Find an outdoor spot where you can see fairly far.

The Exercise

Look at the furthest away object that you can bring into clear focus. Slowly bring you're your gaze in by focusing on closer objects or points of definition (e.g. you could follow a highway line from far to near.) When your focal point is three feet away, lift your forefinger up and gaze at the tip. Slowly move your finger in, continuing to gaze at the tip. Once the fingertip has reached your nose, refocus on your distant object.

Repeat twice.

 This can be done indoors at a window, but you'll be healthier if you get up and go outside!

NEAR FAR 3D   TRACK

Writing On The Wall

This exercise requires you to use your eyes differently than you are used to. It takes some practice, but once you get the hang of it, have some fun with it.

Preparation

Sit or stand in front of a plain white or solid colored wall 10 – 20 feet away.

The Exercise

Without moving your head, use your eyes to "write" on the wall. Start with words that are 4-6 letters long, filling the space available to you. Move to longer or multiple words as you become proficient.

"Write" using cursive letters to reinforce smooth, steady movement of the eyes.

Use your "writing" to stimulate your brain, not just your eyes. Start by writing basic words, but move on to solving math problems, writing haiku, creating anagrams or doing other intellectually stimulating word or number games (that are relatively short).

Indecisive Hitchhiker

Increase eye flexibility while working on peripheral vision.

Preparation

Sit or stand in a relaxed, comfortable position.

The Exercise

Stretch your arms straight out with your thumbs up. Looking straight ahead, move your thumbs apart until just before you lose sight of each thumb with the opposite eye (because your nose gets in the way). If you are looking at 12:00, you're arms should be pointed to approximately 1:00 and 11:00.

Without turning your head, glance back and forth between your thumbs at a moderate pace.

Do this 10-20 times over 1-2 minutes.

 Look at each thumb long enough to bring it into clear focus – don't just glance at it.

UFO Hunter

Two types of eye movements figure prominently in many sports: pursuit and saccadic. Pursuit requires your eyes to follow a target as it moves through space. With saccadic movement, your eyes jump to where you expect a target to be.

Preparation

Stand in a dark or semi-dark room with a flashlight.

Exercise 1 - Pursuit

Run a flashlight over a wall, varying the speed. Holding your head still, follow the light with your eyes as accurately as possible for 2-3 minutes.

Exercise 2 - Saccadic

Switch the flashlight on and off rapidly as you move the light. Still not moving your head, make your eyes jump along the wall to catch each new burst of the flashlight. Again, do this for 2-3 minutes.

 Have someone else move the flashlight so that your eyes don't "pre-track" the light.

30

Study Period

A quick exercise to help your close vision focus.

Preparation

Sit comfortably with some text 10-24 inches away from your eyes.

The Exercise

Find a period at the end of a sentence. Stare at the period while breathing normally. After 30 seconds, use your eyes to trace the inside edge of the period for 10 seconds then to trace the outside edge of the period for 10 seconds. Finish by closing your eyes for another 10 seconds.

Repeat two more times.

 Try doing this with one eye at a time covered (but open). Finish by doing it with both eyes.

Tracing

Develop your peripheral awareness and the ability to focus at all distances. Great for strengthening the link between eyes and brain. Particular benefits for athletes.

Preparation

Find a spot where, without moving your head, you can see at least 10 objects at various distances (near and far) and across the breadth of your field of vision.

The Exercise

Facing forward and without moving your head, trace the edges of 10 different objects with your eyes at a moderate pace.

Keep your eyes moving smoothly the entire time by linking the objects (like you are writing in cursive), then close your eyes for 30 seconds when you are finished.

When you become proficient, start to use objects with more complicated edges. Also try using objects at different distances (branches on a tree to letters in a book).

32

| FLEX | NEAR | FAR | 3D | SIDE | TRACK | | 4 |

Round and Round

Pursuit and saccadic exercise to help see moving objects clearly. Great for sports with a moving ball.

Preparation

Find something that spins freely (an old turntable, bicycle wheel, Lazy Susan, etc.) Print inch high letters of the entire alphabet. Cut and tape them randomly to the perimeter of the "spinner." View from arms length so that you can keep the "spinner" moving.

Exercise 1 - Pursuit

Pick a letter, focus on it and follow it as it spins.

Exercise 2 – Semi-saccadic

Read the letters as they pass a fixed point. Try to keep your focus in one place (e.g. 12:00).

Exercise 3 – Saccadic

Think of a word of at least eight letters. Spell it using the letters on your "spinner" as quickly as possible.

 As you become proficient, make the letters smaller or increase the speed of the "spinner."

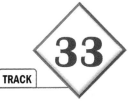

Right-Left Eye Rotation

Stretch and flex each eye independently.

Preparation

Stand or sit comfortably with your back straight, relaxing your shoulders away from your ears.

The Exercise

Place your left palm over your left eye and extend your right arm straight out in front of your right eye. Keeping your head still and focusing on your thumbnail, slowly draw a quarter circle with a 12 inch radius to the right (from clock center to 12:00 to 3:00 to clock center). Blink and follow your thumbnail as it draws the same path in reverse. Next switch your hands and do the same exercise using your left eye while your right eye is covered (this path will be from clock center to 12:00 to 9:00 to clock center.) Repeat the two quarter circles 10 times.

After doing this exercise for a few weeks, start increasing the radius of the quarter circle. Try to work towards a radius of 18-24 inches.

Pen and Cap

Practice using depth perception.

Preparation

Sit comfortably with a pen in one hand and its cap in the other.

The Exercise

Extend your arms to almost full length (keep a slight bend at the elbow). Starting with the cap about a foot over the pen, slowly place the cap on the pen. Make a real effort to judge the depth of both cap and pen – don't try to feel the distance with your arms. Shake your arms out and repeat 10 times.

Once you become proficient, use two pencils and touch their tips or drop a BB into a drinking straw. Also, with every other attempt, bring your hands halfway in to your face.

If you have poor binocular vision and struggle seeing three dimensions, this exercise can at least help you "see" depth better by developing your ability to use perspective as a visual clue.

Mirror Tracking

Train your eyes to track a target when your body is moving.

Preparation

Stand 3-5 feet in front of a mirror and focus on your own eyes.

The Exercise

Focus on your eyes without moving for one minute. While maintaining focus on your eyes, turn your head from side to side and up and down at a moderate pace for another 3-4 minutes. Once this has become a fairly easy process, try it while moving your entire body from side to side.

 Football, basketball, tennis, and baseball are among the sports that require this skill.

 If you are trying to keep your eyes healthy for sports, go out and play catch or go to the batting cage and swing a bat.

Ghost Tracing

Excellent for working on your close vision.

Preparation

Sitting comfortably, hold a Near Eye Chart 10-20 inches in front of you and find the smallest row you can see without straining your eyes.

The Exercise

Keeping your head still, trace the first letter of the row with your eyes. Close your eyes, visualize the same letter, and trace it again. Open your eyes and repeat both steps.

Next, open your eyes and bring the eye chart in until the letters starts to blur. Close your eyes for one deep breath. Open them, focus on the letter, then move the chart back to its original position.

Repeat with at least four letters in the row.

 Inhale with eyes closed, exhale with eyes open.

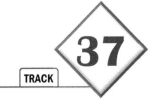

Sideshow

Develop your peripheral awareness. Great for strengthening the link between eyes and brain. Another good exercise for athletes.

Preparation

Sit or stand with a stationary object in front of you and a moving object (such as an oscillating fan or a clock with a second hand) at the edge of your field of vision.

The Exercise

Follow the movement of the item or items in your peripheral field of vision while maintaining your direct focus on the object in front of you. Do this for 1-2 minutes on each side.

As you gain skill and confidence, go to a busy place and follow the passage of people in and out of your peripheral field while you focus on a single point.

Peripheral vision reaches your brain faster than straight-ahead vision.

Colored Dot Drill

A target tracking exercise that is similar to those used by many baseball players.

Preparation

Get a dozen of a single kind of ball (golf balls, lacrosse balls, and baseballs work well.) Use markers of 3-4 different colors to draw a dot on each ball (evenly distributed). Make the dots a half an inch in diameter. Get a partner who is able to toss the balls.

The Exercise

Have your partner randomly select balls and underhand toss them to you from 10-20 feet away. Try to say the color of the dot before catching the ball.

If you're alone, put the balls in a bag so that you can't see them. Pick randomly and toss the ball off a wall.

As you gain proficiency, toss over different distances, increase ball speed, make smaller dots, or use shapes instead of colors.

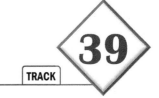

3   3D   TRACK

Peripheral Posts

A peripheral vision exercise that will help with everything from sports to driving.

Preparation

Hold a pencil in each hand 12-18 inches in front of you and about 12 inches apart.

The Exercise

Gaze between the pencils into the distance. Keep your gaze steady with no head movement. Without looking directly at either of the pencils, slowly move the pencils away from each other until they are at the edge of your peripheral vision. Return pencils slowly to the start position. Do this 5-10 times.

Return to the start position and repeat sequence moving one pencil up and the other pencil down. Start with the pencils further apart as you develop proficiency.

Experiment with other movements such as circles, wavy vertical lines, diagonal lines, etc.

40

Toothpicks and Straw

A peripheral vision and depth perception exercise.

Preparation

You will need two drinking straws, two toothpicks and a tall drinking glass. Tape the two straws together so that you have a single straw about 18 inches long. Turn your glass upside down and tape the middle of your "long" straw to the bottom of the glass. Use a marker to make a black line or dot on the tape. Place the glass with straw on a table about 18 inches in front of you with the straw going from side to side.

The Exercise

Sit facing the glass and straw and hold a toothpick in each hand. Focusing on the black line, attempt to put the toothpicks in the straw ends at the same time. Repeat 5-10 times shaking out your arms between each attempt.

Once you become proficient at this, add another straw to make it more difficult. If it is already too hard, use a single straw.

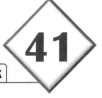

3D | SIDE | TRACK

Eye Massages 1

Not strictly exercises, but these routines will help relax your eyes and your mind.

Preparation

Lie down or sit in a reclined position.

Hot and Cold Compress

Soak one towel in hot water and another in cold. Starting with the hot towel, gently press it to your face, focusing on your eyebrows and closed eyelids. Alternate between the two towels as desired, making sure to end with the cold one.

Full Face Massage

Soak a towel in hot water. Rub your neck and face with the towel, avoiding the eyes. Then, use your fingertips to gently massage your forehead, cheeks, and the perimeter of your closed eyes.

Palm Eye Massage

Close your eyes and very gently rub your eyelids with the palms of your hands in a circular motion. 10 times in each direction should do it.

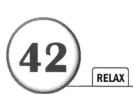

Eye Massages 2

Eyelid Massage

Close your eyes and massage them with circular movements of your fingers for 1-2 minutes. Make sure you press very lightly to avoid damaging your eyes.

Peripheral Acupressure

Starting at the inside corner of the eye, press firmly on the eye sockets. Rotate to a new point every 10 seconds (every five minutes on an imaginary clock). Follow with Light Acupressure.

Light Acupressure

Lightly press three fingers of each hand against your upper eyelids. Hold them there for 1-2 seconds, then release. Repeat five times.

Cool Down

Lean back or lie down with a damp towel placed over your closed eyes.

 Finish every eye workout with "Cool Down" or "Palming."

No Time – Stress Relief

If you're engrossed with work, need to zone out in front of the TV, or are just too tired to give your eyes a workout, at least give your eyes a break.

Preparation

None.

The Exercise

Simply look up from your work/reading/viewing every five minutes or so and focus on something distant and in good light for 5-10 seconds.

Students and those in professions that involve a lot of close work, like tailors, writers and computer operators, are far more likely to be nearsighted than those in active professions like soldiers or police officers.

During close work, your eye muscles contract. If they are contracted for an extended period of time, they can cramp in that position, like when you grip something tightly for an extended period of time then release your grip and have trouble uncurling your fingers.

RELAX   **FAR**   ½

No Time – Flexibility

Do this while standing in line, waiting in traffic, talking on the phone, or even going to the bathroom!

Preparation

None.

The Exercise

1. Look up to your eyebrows.

2. Look down to your mouth.

3. Look to your right ear.

4. Look to your left ear.

5. Roll your eyes in a circle (easiest done by looking at the four corners of the room or an imaginary room). Do it again in the other direction.

6. Finish by looking at the tip of your nose.

No Time – Close Vision

Try these quick movements if you can't find time to do your close vision exercises.

Preparation

None.

Exercise 1

Stop and focus on a single letter of text 10-20 inches away for 20 seconds. Trace the inside and outside edge of the letter. Finish by looking up and focusing on a distant object for a few seconds. Do this every 5-10 minutes while reading or whenever you have a chance if moving about.

Exercise 2

Using a page of text (book, magazine, newspaper, etc.), jump from period to period down the entire page. Pause long enough to trace the edge of each period before allowing your eyes to jump to the next period. A single page should allow you to hit 10-20 periods.

Do this 3-5 times a day.

46

No Time – Distance

On days when you can't follow your routine, use this easy exercise to practice your distance seeing.

Preparation

None.

The Exercise

Consciously focus on distant objects without straining your eyes as you go about your daily routine.

You will almost always be able to find something to focus on, but examples include:

- Read road signs and license plate numbers when you are driving (don't just ignore the details like you do most days),

- Watch birds in flight or airplanes in the sky,

- Count stars or lit windows (if in the city) at night,

- Track the ball at a soccer game or focus on a hockey players skates, or

- Trace the branches of a tree in winter or find them amongst the leaves the rest of the year.

No Time – Peripheral

Do this exercise while walking to help your peripheral awareness.

Preparation

Walk on a flat surface.

The Exercise

While looking straight ahead, first take a few seconds to notice the condition of the sky (sunny, white fluffy clouds, overcast, etc.) then take a few seconds to make yourself aware of the surface you are walking on (stone, brick, dirt, moving sidewalk, etc.).

Finish by identifying objects on both your right and left, while continuing to focus straight ahead.

Even though you may already know the weather, what you are walking on, or what you are walking past, double check using your peripheral vision. Notice the color or the texture – whatever helps you make the visual connection.

Try to do this five times over the course of the day.

Appendix 1
Vision tests and progress tracking

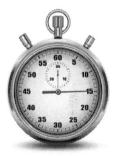

Vision Tests & Progress Tracking

If you want to determine whether or not your vision is improving, the following tests will give you a baseline and consistent means for tracking any improvement. Do only those that you need or care about.

I suggest running through the tests once every 3-4 weeks. It is more important to do your exercises regularly than it is to take the tests. For many of us, however, the regularity of test are motivation to do the exercises. 3-4 weeks is long enough to allow for some progress, but not long enough to let you get away with slacking off for too many days.

Feel free to adjust the tests according to your environmental constraints. The size and space in your home will dictate how and where you do your Distance Test. Your ability to get someone to help you will affect how you do the tracking test. Just keep three things in mind when doing the tests:

1. Use common sense – do the Distance Test from further away, do the Close Vision Test as close as you can. Not rocket science here!

2. Be consistent – testing yourself over many months is useless if you don't do the test the same way every time.

3. Don't cheat – telling yourself that you can see something clearly when you can't or guessing at what you see and happening to get it right is not helpful. Have some respect for the person you'd be cheating.

A tracking template for these tests is included here and a larger version can be found at www.the15minutefix.com.

The 15 Minute Fix: VISION

Vision Improvement Tracking

Start Date: _____

Test			Date:																
1	Close Vision Test 1	Left	Line #																
		Right																	
		Center																	
2	Close Vision Test 2	Left	Inches																
		Right																	
		Center																	
3	Distance Vision Test	Left	#/Inches																
		Right																	
		Center																	
4	Depth Perception Test 1	Overall success	Scale 1-5																
		Right strength																	
		Left strength																	
		2 Fingers	2 Dots	Scale 1-5																
		Overall success																	
		Right strength																	
		Left strength																	
5	Depth Perception Test 2	Pass 1	Straws																
		Pass 2																	
		Pass 3																	
6	Peripheral Vision Test 1	Right	Inches																
		Left																	
7	Peripheral Vision Test 2	Right	Inches																
		Left																	
8	Sports Vision Test	Pass 1	Balls																
		Pass 2																	
		Pass 3																	

Close Vision Test 1

This test will help you track any improvement in your ability to read small print at close range.

Preparation

Select three Near Vision Eye Charts at random. Place them in a stack where you can see them (tacked to a wall, propped on your desk, held – anything you can do every time you do the test). To avoid cheating yourself, keep the charts at arm length while setting up. Using a tape measure, move your head such that the tip of your nose is 14 inches from the charts.

The Test

Starting with your left hand over your left eye, use your right eye to read the line with the smallest print that you can still see in clear focus. Record the line number. Remove the top eye chart and repeat using your left eye. Then, with the last chart, repeat using both eyes.

Acclimate your eyes for this and every eye test, by making sure that you have been in the room where you are doing the test (or similar light conditions) for at least 10 minutes.

NEAR

Close Vision Test 2

This test will help you track how close in you are able to read text. Do this after Close Vision Test 1.

Preparation

Use the same Near Vision Eye Charts that you used in Close Vision Test 1. Place them in the same order at arms length (taped to a wall or propped on a table or desk – something that will leave a hand free so that you can make the final measurement.) To avoid cheating yourself, keep the charts at arm length while setting up. You will need a flexible tape measure too.

The Test

Covering your left eye, focus your right eye on the eye chart line that you selected in Close Vision Test 1 (1ˢᵗ pass). Slowly move your face toward the eye chart. Stop at the point where you lose clear focus of the letters in your selected eye chart line. Without moving your head, use the tape measure to determine the distance between the tip of your nose and the chart.

Repeat the test using your left eye, then both eyes.

Record all three results.

NEAR

Distance Vision Test

This test will help you track your ability to see clearly at a distance.

Preparation

Find a space in your home where you can stand at least 30 feet from a wall (with an unimpeded view and no obstacles in front of you). The first time you do this test, mark a spot on the floor around 30 feet from the wall. You will want to use this mark every time you do this test. Select three Far Vision Eye Charts at random. Tape the charts side by side on the wall or prop them on a table against the wall. Try to avoid reading the eye chart while setting up. A tape measure will help.

The Test

Standing at your 30 foot mark, cover your left eye and look at the right eye chart. Determine the highest line you cannot see clearly. (This should be consistent from test to test, although if your distance vision improves, you may eventually drop down a line.) Walk forward until you can read that line clearly. Measure and record the distance from your starting point.

Repeat using your left eye with the left chart and both eyes with the center chart.

FAR

Depth Perception Test 1

This test will help you assess your binocular vision.

Preparation

While sitting, position the black dot below in front of your face (on a table or desk) a full arm length away.

The Test

While focusing on the dot, hold your finger between your eyes and the dot, about eight inches from your nose. You should see two fingers on either side of the dot.

Now focus on the finger. You should see two dots on either side of your finger.

Record on a scale of 1-5 your ability to do this exercise and the strength of the double images. You are looking to reach a point where you see the double image automatically (a 5), and you see the double images equally. This is a difficult test to track, but with time, you'll know if you are improving.

3D

Depth Perception Test 2

This test will help you track any improvement in your depth perception.

Preparation

You will need 10 toothpicks and an object that is roughly 12x12 inches into which you can stick them (piece of Styrofoam, cardboard, etc.). Stick the toothpicks in your object, arbitrarily distributed and standing up straight. Place the object with toothpicks on a flat surface such that you can comfortably sit or stand and be at eye level with it. You will also need five straight drinking straws cut in half (10 pieces).

The Test

With the foremost toothpicks about 12 inches in front of you and at eye level, take a straw and hold it about a millimeter above one of the toothpicks. (If you touch the toothpick with the straw, move to another toothpick and come back to that one later.) Try to drop it on the toothpick. Repeat with the remaining straws and toothpicks. Try to skip around rather than simply moving to an adjacent toothpick. Record how many stayed upright on a toothpick. Take two more passes, recording each.

Peripheral Vision Test 1

This test will help you track any improvement in your peripheral awareness.

Preparation

Sit at a table that is wider than your arm span (both arms stretched out to the side). Sit with your torso against the table and your chin over the edge of the table. Stretch your arms out and place a ruler (or, better yet, a yardstick) under each hand in a manner that will allow you to measure the distance from the edge of the table.

The Test

Stretch your arms out to full length and stick your thumbs up in the air. Looking straight ahead, pull your arms back so that you can not see your thumbs. Focus on something straight in front of you and move your thumbs in until you can see them. Drop your hands to the table and measure their distance to the edge of the table.

6

SIDE

Peripheral Vision Test 2

This test will help you track any improvement in your peripheral vision.

Preparation

This is done the same way as Peripheral Vision Test 1, except that you will need some pieces of paper with individual letters at least one inch high (printable one inch high letters can be found at www.the15minutefix.com). Shuffle and place your letters face down on the table.

The Test

Without looking at the letters, take one in each hand. Stretch your arms out to full length and looking straight ahead, pull your arms back so that you can not see the letters (which you can now hold up). Focus on something straight in front of you and move your hands in until you can identify each letter. Drop your hands to the table and measure their distance to the edge of the table.

 None of these tests are meant to substitute for a professional eye examination. They are for tracking and informational purposes only.

Sports Vision Test

This test (essentially the Colored Dot Drill) will help you monitor any progress in your ability to track moving objects.

Preparation

Get a dozen of a single kind of ball (golf balls, lacrosse balls, or baseballs work well). Use markers of 3-4 different colors to draw a dot on each ball (evenly distributed). Make the dots a half an inch in diameter. Get a partner who can toss the balls to you.

The Test

Have your partner randomly select 10 balls and toss them to you from 10 feet away. Say the color of the dot before catching the ball. Record how many you got right. Repeat two more times and record. Try to use the same partner each time you do the test – this will help you keep the speed and arc of the toss consistent from test to test.

If you reach the point where this or any other test is getting too easy, don't be afraid to make it harder – just do it in a way that you can track consistently from test to test.

Appendix 2
Workout template and sample plans

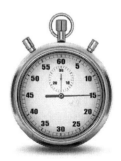

Workout Template and Sample Plans

Tracking your progress should be simple – otherwise you'll probably stop doing it. You only need a couple of basic pieces of information to draw conclusions. However, these often vary from exercise to exercise, so the trick is to use a tracking mechanism that informs and motivates you without becoming burdensome in its own right. The best way to do this is to plan your workouts in advance. As I discussed in the Introduction, I suggest planning your routine in three stages:

- Start with one or two warm-up and circulation exercises,

- Structure the body of your routine around areas of particular concern, and

- Finish with at least one *Relaxation* exercise and one *Flexibility* exercise.

In the following pages, you will find a generic blank template that can be used to design your own weekly routine, along with some sample plans that you can use to get started. The sample plans can also be used to help you generate ideas for your own routine. Many of the sample plans are focused on a single vision concern, so I would urge you to combine two or three of them. You might pick two of them and alternate weeks or even switch between them on a daily basis.

When developing your own routine, first consider your goals. You might want to work on peripheral vision, see better over long distances, or simply have better overall health. Each of these goals will lead toward a different exercise plan. Having multiple goals will complicate things even more. Therefore, I suggest that you find all of the exercises that are consistent with your goals and begin to experiment with them. If there are too many to do in a day, spread them out over as many days as is necessary, mixed in with some warm-up and all-over exercises. You'll figure out fairly quickly which exercises work for you. Make these the main part of your workouts. Eliminate those that are too easy, too hard, or simply unpleasant. You can always bring them back in later, when you need to add variety to your workout.

Now think about your environmental and time constraints. Here are some ways you might think about structuring your routine:

- If you can set aside at least 15 minutes a day, in a single block, do 4-8 exercises from your routine each day, mixing them up as you go along.

- If you're going to have trouble doing exercises every day, try fitting more of your exercises into a 20-25 minute block that you do 3-4 times a week. On your off days, do one or more of the "No Time" exercises or a Relaxation/Stress Relief exercise.

- If you can't carve out any significant blocks of time, focus on exercises you can do given your particular lifestyle constraints and fit them in during the free moments in your day – even if those moments are brief. This may mean that you only do the "anytime, anyplace" exercises during the week, saving a few more involved exercises for the weekends.

Play around with your routine. Figure out through experimentation which exercises and what schedule works best for you. Tracking your exercises as you experiment is vital to the process of finding good routines.

Once you settle on a general routine, keeping a tracking sheet handy will help you remember to do your exercises, stay motivated, and know when exercises are getting stale and need to be switched up. It is too easy to lose track if you don't write it down.

The workout samples that follow are:

1. Stress Relief

2. Eye Flexibility

3. Close Vision

4. Distance Vision

5. Depth Perception

6. Peripheral Vision

7. Tracking/Sports

8. Desk Workout

9. On The Go

Keep in mind that the templates are limited by the size of the page and may not suit your particular lifestyle. Each of the templates has nine exercises, but you may want a rotation that includes 12, 15, or 20 exercises. In addition to the templates and sample plans that follow, www.the15minutefix.com has a variety of larger and more diversified templates and sample plans. You will also find templates that can be downloaded and edited to your specifications.

The 15 Minute Fix

Workout Title: _____   **Week of:** _____

Exercise	Times/Day		Sun	Mon	Tue	Wed	Thus	Fri	Sat
		Time E/A*							
		Reps/Sets							
		Notes							
		Time E/A							
		Reps/Sets							
		Notes							
		Time E/A							
		Reps/Sets							
		Notes							
		Time E/A							
		Reps/Sets							
		Notes							
		Time E/A							
		Reps/Sets							
		Notes							
		Time E/A							
		Reps/Sets							
		Notes							
		Time E/A							
		Reps/Sets							
		Notes							
		Time E/A							
		Reps/Sets							
		Notes							
		Time E/A							
		Reps/Sets							
		Notes							
		Time E/A							
		Reps/Sets							
		Notes							
		Time E/A							

* estimated/actual

Total Weekly Time
Average Time per Day

◯ The 15 Minute Fix: VISION **Workout Title: STRESS RELIEF SAMPLE** Week of: _____

Exercise	Times/Day		Sun	Mon	Tue	Wed	Thus	Fri	Sat
1	1	Time E/A	3 /	3 /	3 /	3 /	3 /	3 /	3 /
5x5 Warm-up		Reps/Sets	/	/	/	/	/	/	/
		Notes							
7	1	Time E/A	3 /	/	/	3 /	/	/	/
Phantom Sight		Reps/Sets	/	/	/	/	/	/	/
		Notes							
6	1	Time E/A	5 /	/	/	5 /	/	/	5 /
Relaxed Eyes		Reps/Sets	/	/	/	/	/	/	/
		Notes							
4	1	Time E/A	/	3 /	/	/	3 /	/	/
Sleepy Eyes		Reps/Sets	/	/	/	/	/	/	/
		Notes							
8	1	Time E/A	/	4 /	/	/	4 /	/	4 /
Visualization		Reps/Sets	/	/	/	/	/	/	/
		Notes							
42	1	Time E/A	/	5 /	/	/	5 /	/	/
Eye Massages 1		Reps/Sets	/	/	/	/	/	/	/
		Notes							
9	1	Time E/A	/	/	3 /	/	/	3 /	3 /
Rolling in the Dark		Reps/Sets	/	/	/	/	/	/	/
		Notes							
17	1	Time E/A	/	/	5 /	/	/	5 /	/
Trataka		Reps/Sets	/	/	/	/	/	/	/
		Notes							
43	1	Time E/A	/	/	5 /	/	/	5 /	/
Eye Massages 2		Reps/Sets	/	/	/	/	/	/	/
		Notes							
		Time E/A	11 /	15 /	16 /	11 /	15 /	16 /	15 /

Total Weekly Time	99 /
Average Time per Day	14.1 /

Exercise	Times/Day		Sun	Mon	Tue	Wed	Thus	Fri	Sat
1 — 5x5 Warm-up	1	Time E/A	3		3		3		
		Reps/Sets							
		Notes							
9 — Rolling In the Dark	1	Time E/A	3		3		3		
		Reps/Sets							
		Notes							
12 — Compass Points	1	Time E/A	2		2		2		
		Reps/Sets							
		Notes							
28 — Writing On The Wall	1	Time E/A	3		3		3		
		Reps/Sets							
		Notes							
14 — Steady Gaze	1	Time E/A	5		5		5		
		Reps/Sets							
		Notes							
20 — Figure Eight	1	Time E/A	3		3		3		
		Reps/Sets							
		Notes							
24 — Text Trombone	1	Time E/A	5		5		5		
		Reps/Sets							
		Notes							
34 — Right-Left Eye Rotation	1	Time E/A	3		3		3		
		Reps/Sets							
		Notes							
45 — No Time – Flexibility	3	Time E/A		9		9		9	
		Reps/Sets							
		Notes							
		Time E/A	27	9	27	9	27	9	0

Total Weekly Time   108

Average Time per Day   15.4

○— The 15 Minute Fix: VISION   **Workout Title: CLOSE VISION SAMPLE**   **Week of:** _____

Exercise		Times/Day		Sun	Mon	Tue	Wed	Thus	Fri	Sat
1	5x5 Warm-up	1	Time E/A	3	3	3	3	3	3	3
			Reps/Sets							
			Notes							
11	Rockin'	1	Time E/A	2			2			
			Reps/Sets							
			Notes							
25	Pencil Focus	1	Time E/A	4			4			
			Reps/Sets							
			Notes							
21	Simple Trombone	1	Time E/A		3			3		
			Reps/Sets							
			Notes							
31	Study Period	1	Time E/A		3			3		
			Reps/Sets							
			Notes							
15	Near-Far	1	Time E/A			3			3	
			Reps/Sets							
			Notes							
37	Ghost Tracing	1	Time E/A			3			3	
			Reps/Sets							
			Notes							
23	Complex Trombone	1	Time E/A							10
			Reps/Sets							
			Notes							
3	Palming	1	Time E/A	4	4	4	4	4	4	4
			Reps/Sets							
			Notes							
			Time E/A	13	13	13	13	13	13	17

Total Weekly Time   95
Average Time per Day   13.6

The 15 Minute Fix: VISION

Workout Title: DISTANCE VISION SAMPLE

Week of: _____

Exercise		Times/Day		Sun	Mon	Tue	Wed	Thus	Fri	Sat
1	5x5 Warm-up	1	Time E/A	3		3		3		
			Reps/Sets							
			Notes							
13	Distance Focusing	1	Time E/A	3		3		3		
			Reps/Sets							
			Notes							
15	Near-Far	1	Time E/A	3		3		3		
			Reps/Sets							
			Notes							
26	Telescoping	1	Time E/A	2		2		2		
			Reps/Sets							
			Notes							
27	Distant to Close	1	Time E/A	2		2		2		
			Reps/Sets							
			Notes							
32	Tracing	1	Time E/A	4		4		4		
			Reps/Sets							
			Notes							
3	Palming	1	Time E/A	4		4		4		
			Reps/Sets							
			Notes							
5	Blinking	2	Time E/A		4		4		4	
			Reps/Sets							
			Notes							
47	No Time – Distance	5	Time E/A		5		5		5	
			Reps/Sets							
			Notes							
			Time E/A	21	9	21	9	21	9	0

Total Weekly Time	90
Average Time per Day	12.9

The 15 Minute Fix: VISION

Workout Title: DEPTH PERCEPTION SAMPLE   **Week of:**

Exercise		Times/Day		Sun	Mon	Tue	Wed	Thus	Fri	Sat
1	5x5 Warm-up	1	Time E/A	3 /	3 /	3 /	3 /	3 /	3 /	3 /
			Reps/Sets							
			Notes							
11	Rockin'	1	Time E/A	2 /	/	2 /	/	2 /	/	/
			Reps/Sets							
			Notes							
25	Pencil Focus	1	Time E/A	4 /	/	4 /	/	4 /	/	/
			Reps/Sets							
			Notes							
35	Pen and Cap	1	Time E/A	2 /	/	2 /	/	2 /	/	/
			Reps/Sets							
			Notes							
21	Simple Trombone	1	Time E/A	/	3 /	/	3 /	/	3 /	/
			Reps/Sets							
			Notes							
27	Distant to Close	1	Time E/A	/	2 /	/	2 /	/	2 /	/
			Reps/Sets							
			Notes							
41	Toothpicks and Straw	1	Time E/A	/	3 /	/	3 /	/	3 /	/
			Reps/Sets							
			Notes							
17	Trataka	1	Time E/A	/	/	/	/	/	/	5 /
			Reps/Sets							
			Notes							
3	Palming	1	Time E/A	4 /	4 /	4 /	4 /	4 /	4 /	4 /
			Reps/Sets							
			Notes							
			Time E/A	15 /	15 /	15 /	15 /	15 /	15 /	12 /

Total Weekly Time 102 /
Average Time per Day 14.6 /

The 15 Minute Fix: VISION

Workout Title: PERIPHERAL VISION SAMPLE

Week of: _____

Exercise	Times/Day		Sun	Mon	Tue	Wed	Thus	Fri	Sat
1	1	Time E/A	3	3	3	3	3	3	
5x5 Warm-up		Reps/Sets							
		Notes							
18	1	Time E/A	2		2		2		
Four Corners		Reps/Sets							
		Notes							
40	1	Time E/A	2		2		2		
Peripheral Posts		Reps/Sets							
		Notes							
20	1	Time E/A	3		3		3		
Figure Eight		Reps/Sets							
		Notes							
29	1	Time E/A	2		2		2		
Indecisive Hitchhiker		Reps/Sets							
		Notes							
19	1	Time E/A		3		3		3	
Big Ben		Reps/Sets							
		Notes							
33	1	Time E/A		3		3		3	
Round and Round		Reps/Sets							
		Notes							
38	1	Time E/A		3		3		3	
Slideshow		Reps/Sets							
		Notes							
3	1	Time E/A	4	4	4	4	4	4	
Palming		Reps/Sets							
		Notes							
		Time E/A	16	16	16	16	16	16	0

Total Weekly Time 96

Average Time per Day 13.7

The 15 Minute Fix: VISION   **Workout Title: TRACKING/SPORTS SAMPLE**   Week of: _____

Exercise	Times/Day		Sun	Mon	Tue	Wed	Thus	Fri	Sat
1 — 5x5 Warm-up	1	Time E/A	3	3	3	3	3	3	3
		Reps/Sets							
		Notes							
32 — Tracing	1	Time E/A	4		4		4		
		Reps/Sets							
		Notes							
38 — Slideshow	1	Time E/A	3		3		3		
		Reps/Sets							
		Notes							
40 — Peripheral Posts	1	Time E/A							
		Reps/Sets		2		2		2	
		Notes							
36 — Mirror Tracking	1	Time E/A							
		Reps/Sets		5		5		5	
		Notes							
33 — Round and Round	1	Time E/A							3
		Reps/Sets							
		Notes							
39 — Colored Dot Drill	1	Time E/A							3
		Reps/Sets							
		Notes							
30 — UFO Hunter	1	Time E/A							5
		Reps/Sets							
		Notes							
3 — Palming	1	Time E/A	4	4	4	4	4	4	4
		Reps/Sets							
		Notes							
		Time E/A	14	14	14	14	14	14	18

Total Weekly Time: 102

Average Time per Day: 14,6

Workout Title: DESK WORKOUT SAMPLE

Week of: _____

Exercise		Times/Day		Sun	Mon	Tue	Wed	Thus	Fri	Sat
5	Blinking	3	Time E/A		6 /	6 /	6 /	6 /	6 /	/
			Reps/Sets	/	/	/	/	/	/	/
			Notes							
4	Sleepy Eyes	1	Time E/A		3 /	/	3 /	/	3 /	/
			Reps/Sets	/	/	/	/	/	/	/
			Notes							
12	Compass Points	1	Time E/A		2 /	/	2 /	/	2 /	/
			Reps/Sets	/	/	/	/	/	/	/
			Notes							
10	Eye Squeeze	1	Time E/A		/	3 /	/	3 /	/	/
			Reps/Sets	/	/	/	/	/	/	/
			Notes							
14	Steady Gaze	1	Time E/A		/	5 /	/	5 /	/	/
			Reps/Sets	/	/	/	/	/	/	/
			Notes							
19	Big Ben	1	Time E/A		3 /	3 /	3 /	3 /	/	/
			Reps/Sets	/	/	/	/	/	/	/
			Notes							
13	Distance Focusing	1	Time E/A		/	/	/	/	/	/
			Reps/Sets	/	/	/	/	/	/	/
			Notes							
20	Figure Eight	1	Time E/A		3 /	/	/	/	3 /	/
			Reps/Sets	/	/	/	/	/	/	/
			Notes							
2	20-20-20	8	Time E/A		4 /	4 /	4 /	4 /	4 /	/
			Reps/Sets	/	/	/	/	/	/	/
			Notes							
			Time E/A	0 /	21 /	21 /	18 /	21 /	21 /	0 /

Total Weekly Time 102

Average Time per Day 14.6

The 15 Minute Fix: VISION

Workout Title: ON THE GO SAMPLE

Week of: _____

Exercise	Times/Day		Sun	Mon	Tue	Wed	Thus	Fri	Sat
5 Blinking	4	Time E/A		8	8		8	8	
		Reps/Sets							
		Notes							
14 Steady Gaze	1	Time E/A		5			5		
		Reps/Sets							
		Notes							
27 Distant to Close	1	Time E/A		2			2		
		Reps/Sets							
		Notes							
38 Sideshow	1	Time E/A		3			3		
		Reps/Sets							
		Notes							
12 Compass Points	1	Time E/A		2			2		
		Reps/Sets							
		Notes							
32 Tracing	1	Time E/A			4			4	
		Reps/Sets							
		Notes							
13 Distance Focusing	1	Time E/A			3			3	
		Reps/Sets							
		Notes							
26 Telescoping	1	Time E/A			2			2	
		Reps/Sets							
		Notes							
10 Eye Squeeze	2	Time E/A		6	6		6	6	
		Reps/Sets							
		Notes							
		Time E/A	0	26	23	0	26	23	0

Total Weekly Time 98

Average Time per Day 14.0

Appendix 3
Eye Charts

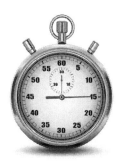

Near and Far Eye Charts

The following eye charts can be used for the vision tests and the exercises that suggest using them. They are based on Snellen Eye Charts which are commonly used by ophthalmologists and other eye care professionals to measure visual acuity.

Larger eye charts and more letter combinations can be downloaded and printed from www.the15minutefix.com. (The web site also has printable letters which can be utilized in Exercise 33 and Vision Test 7.)

These charts are not meant to be used as a substitute for an examination and assessment by a trained eye specialist. As such, they may not adhere to standardized fonts, size, etc. The key, for our purposes here, is for you to be consistent in your use of the charts, particularly for self-tests. Whether you are using charts in this book or eBook, charts downloaded from www.the15minutefix.com, charts you have made, or charts you have found elsewhere, use the same type of chart each time.

Far Eye Chart 1

1   **EN**

2   **DTL**

3   **PNCO**

4   **FDPZC**

5   **LOEPTF**

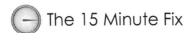 The 15 Minute Fix

1 **FP**

2 **TOZ**

3 **LPEN**

4 **PECFD**

5 **NDFCZP**

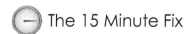 The 15 Minute Fix

1 ZC

2 NLO

3 PDFE

4 ZNECT

5 LPODZF

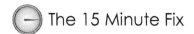 The 15 Minute Fix

1 **PE**

2 **ZOL**

3 **CFTD**

4 **EDNTO**

5 **ZFCPLN**

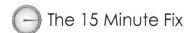

The 15 Minute Fix

1   **NP**

2   **OTE**

3   **LCFD**

4   **PNZFT**

5   **DCFZOP**

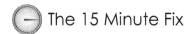

1 **DZ**

2 **POL**

3 **CEFN**

4 **TCPDO**

5 **NEFDLT**

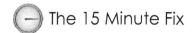 The 15 Minute Fix

Near Eye Chart 1

1   L C Z E P T F D O

2   C O D T N L E P Z F

3   P F N E C Z O T D L

4   F O T D L E P N Z C

5   E N D L T O Z C F P

6   L P C F E T N O D Z

7   P E Z O L C F T D N

8   D E F P O T Z N C E

9   T F N D O P Z L E C

10   F E L O P N Z D T C

11   E D Y N L C O P E N

The 15 Minute Fix

Near Eye Chart 2

1 E N D L T O Z C F

2 L P C F E T N O D Z

3 P E Z O L C F T D N

4 D E F P O T Z N C E

5 T F N D O P Z L E C

6 F E L O P N Z D T C

7 Z D T N L C O P E N

8 L C Z E P T F D O N

9 C O D T N L E P Z F

10 P F N E C Z O T D L

11 F O T D L E P N C

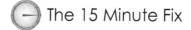 The 15 Minute Fix

Near Eye Chart 3

1   E O P Z T L C D F

2   T D P C F Z O N E L

3   N D Z E L C F O T P

4   P T L F N C Z D E O

5   C F D T E O P L N Z

6   L N D C Z O T E P F

7   Z P T O D N E C F L

8   C T F N E D Z O L P

9   L C P T Z D F E O N

10   Z O E C F L D P N T

11   E T O L N F D C E P

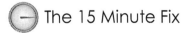 The 15 Minute Fix

Near Eye Chart 4

1   L N D C Z O T E P

2   Z P T O D N E C F L

3   C T F N E D Z O L P

4   L C P T Z D F E O N

5   Z O E C F L D P N T

6   E T O L N F D C Z P

7   O P Z E T L C D F N

8   T D P C F Z O N E L

9   N D Z E L C F O T P

10   P T L F N C Z D E O

11   O F D T Z O P L N E

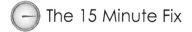 The 15 Minute Fix

Near Eye Chart 5

1 **P E L N O T D Z F**

2 **C L P O T D Z E N F**

3 **T F P L D E O Z C N**

4 **Z E P F O N D C T L**

5 **P F C Z D O N E T L**

6 **L T F P O N C Z E D**

7 **D C L F O Z P E N T**

8 **N F O E P Z C D L T**

9 **T L Z D C P O F N E**

10 **C L P O T D Z E N F**

11 **N D T F C L O Z E F**

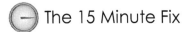 The 15 Minute Fix

Near Eye Chart 6

1   **T L Z D C P O F N**

2   **D C L F O Z P E N T**

3   **L D T O Z N E C F P**

4   **C Z N P E D O F L T**

5   **L C O D E F Z N P T**

6   **P E L N O T D Z F C**

7   Z O T N C D F E P L

8   T F P L D E O Z C N

9   Z E P F O N D C T L

10   T C O L D Z E N P F

11   N F O E P Z C D L T

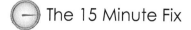 The 15 Minute Fix

Appendix 4
Tips for taking care of your eyes

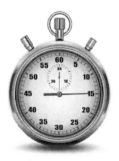

Taking Care Of Your Eyes

- Make sure you have regular eye exams.

- Avoid touching your eyes, and if you do rub around your eyes, make sure your hands are clean.

- Do not apply heavy pressure to your eyes.

- Blink a lot!

- Stay hydrated, give your body the proper nutrients it needs, and get enough sleep.

- If you have allergies, see a specialist to make sure you are managing them well. Allergies can irritate eyes, leading you to rub them.

- If your eyes tend to become dry, get some preservative free artificial tear eye drops.

- Improve your indoor air quality. If you have dry eyes, use a humidifier and lower the thermostat.

- Don't sleep with eye makeup on – get it <u>all</u> off.

- Make sure your eyes get exposed to indirect sunlight every day (just make sure you never look directly at the sun).

- Use, but don't overuse, sunglasses. Use them only when necessary and make sure they block out 99 to 100 percent of both UV-A and UV-B radiation.

- Use appropriate eye protection when working with tools or chemicals or when engaged in activities that could damage eyes. Be aware that eyeglasses are not safety glasses – they may not suit all activities.

- In particular, avoid exposure to gases like ammonia, chlorine, and formaldehyde, as they cause serious eye irritation, and organic solvents, which can damage vision.

- If you have glasses or contacts, use them.

- If you use a CRT computer monitor, switch to a flat-panel monitor or at least use an antiglare filter.

- Wear your seatbelt.

- Stop smoking and try to avoid second-hand smoke.

Appendix 5
Good reading habits

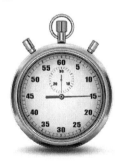

Good Reading Habits

Reading is one of the great things that our eyes make possible, but it can also be one of the most strenuous activities for our eyes. Especially since so much of our reading is at work where we can't choose our lighting or at the end of the day when we are exhausted.

Personally, I find it difficult to enforce good reading habits on myself (I often read in bed, when I am tired, and with insufficient light), so I try to improve my eyes in other ways, particularly through eye exercises. Nevertheless, you may find that following a few of these tips may help relieve some eye strain, improve your retention or help you stay awake while you read.

- Do not read when tired or sick. Reading when you are struggling to keep your eyes open strains them. If you find that you are falling asleep, re-reading words or forgetting what you just read, put the book down.

- Maintain a good posture while reading. Keep your back and neck erect while holding your text in front of you. This will maximize blood flow to your head and eyes. It's also good for the rest of you.

- Every five minutes focus on a single letter for 5-10 seconds, then focus on a distant object for another 5-10 seconds.

- Don't read for more than 30 minutes without taking a break. Stand up, take deep breaths (fresh air if you can), and practice your distance focusing.

- Read in good bright light. Natural sunlight is the best, but if that is not available read near a 100-150 watt light source.

- If you are using a CRT monitor with your computer, replace it with a flat screen monitor or print out anything longer than a couple of paragraphs.

Appendix 6
Food that is
good for your eyes

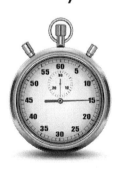

Food that is good for your eyes

The foods covered in this appendix are not only good for your eyes but, as part of a balanced, healthy diet, are also great for your overall health. I have broken them into groups generally based on the specific nutrients that are good for your eyes. I highly recommend you get your nutrients through high quality food sources rather than through supplements. Also remember, the fresher and more natural the food, the higher the levels of nutrients.

Antioxidants:

Anthocyanin – An antioxidant that may improve night vision.

Glutathione – An important antioxidant for the lens of the eye and many other parts of the body. Glutathione also helps in the proper utilization of other nutrients such as vitamins C and E.

Lutein and zeaxanthin – Found in high concentrations in the eye, including the lens, retina, and macula, these two antioxidants absorb 40 to 90 percent of blue light intensity, acting like sunscreen for your eyes. Studies have shown that eating foods rich in lutein and zeaxanthin can increase the pigment density in the macula — and greater pigment density means better retina protection and a lower risk of macular degeneration.

Lycopene – A carotenoid that can help promote good vision.

Vitamin A/Beta Carotene – Beta carotene is an antioxidant that helps reduce the risk of macular degeneration and cataracts. The body converts beta carotene into vitamin A, which boosts cell and tissue regeneration, with particular benefit to the eye lens. Since vitamin A is stored in the liver for future use, 20 mg of beta carotene is plenty. You can get this from a single cup of carrot juice or two cups of spinach.

Vitamin C – An antioxidant shown specifically to protect the eyes. Remember, the best way to get this vitamin, which helps your body produce collagen, is to consume it via natural sources.

Vitamin E – Another antioxidant that is critical in eye care and may also slow macular degeneration and decrease risk of cataracts.

These foods are some of the best sources of eye-friendly antioxidants:

Apricots – Apricots are a good source of beta carotene and lycopene.

Bell peppers, broccoli, and Brussels sprouts – Tons of vitamin C & E and effective in boosting glutathione.

Berries – One of the top sources of antioxidants, including anthocyanin and vitamin C, berries appear to play an important role in decreasing cancer risks, cardiovascular disease, and Alzheimer's disease. Studies have also found the antioxidants in berries reduce the risk of macular degeneration, cataracts, and other eyes diseases.

Carrots – Loaded with beta carotene.

Chicken – The best animal source for lycopene. Try to

use natural, organic, or local chicken. Many large scale producers of chicken bathe the meat in chlorine and other chemicals, lowering much of its nutritional value.

Citrus fruits – The gold standard for vitamin C! Oranges and grapefruits are the best sources.

Dark grapes, cherries, and dark plums – Good sources of anthocyanin. To get the most benefit, eat the peel too.

Garlic and onions – Help your body boost glutathione levels.

Milk – Milk is usually fortified with vitamin A. It is also a good source of riboflavin and can help reduce your risk of cataracts. Choose low-fat milk over whole milk to keep the saturated fat low and prevent plaque buildup in the eyes' blood vessels. Cheese, eggs, and liver are also good sources of vitamin A.

Red fruits and vegetables – Anything red such as red peppers, red cabbage, beets, watermelon, and pink grapefruit is likely a good source of anthocyanin and lycopene. If you don't like red veggies, try asparagus.

Spinach, kale, and collard greens – Provide four eye-protecting ingredients, including vitamin C, beta carotene and large amounts of lutein and zeaxanthin. These are also high in sulfur which aids glutathione production.

Sweet potatoes – More beta carotene and vitamin E!

Tomatoes – The best source of lycopene. To get the most lycopene out of your tomatoes, cook them. Tomatoes also help glutathione production.

Wheat Germ – A top source of vitamin E.

Whole grains and nuts – Sunflower seeds and almonds in particular have a lot of vitamin E.

Omega-3 fatty acids – Studies have shown that regularly eating foods rich in omega-3 fats can help protect tiny blood vessels buried within the eyes and may reduce the risk of macular degeneration and dry eye syndrome. Essential fatty acids also may promote proper drainage of intraocular fluid from the eye, lowering the risk of high eye pressure and glaucoma.

The best sources of omega-3 fatty acids include:

Cold water fatty fishes – These include: sardines, salmon, mackerel, tuna, and anchovies. Wild fish has significantly higher levels of omega-3 fatty acids (and other beneficial nutrients) than farm raised fish. Fish is by far the best source of omega-3 fats.

Nuts – If you don't like fish, walnuts, flaxseed, tofu, and canola and soybean oils are decent non-fish sources of alpha-linolenic acid which the body converts to omega-3 fatty acids.

Zinc – Zinc deficiency has been linked to impaired vision, poor night vision, and cloudy cataracts. Found in the retina, zinc helps the functioning of enzymes responsible for eye health. In people with macular degeneration, levels of zinc in the retina can be very low, so eating zinc-rich foods is a logical first step for preventing and treating macular degeneration. Zinc also helps the body absorb antioxidants and fight disease.

Foods rich in zinc include:

Eggs – Also a good source of lutein and vitamin A and, if enriched, omega-3 fatty acids.

<u>Lean beef</u> – Choose lean cuts to reduce the overall saturated fat in your diet.

<u>Ostrich</u> – A healthy and delicious lean substitute for any red or white meat. Look for it in specialty stores or online. In addition to zinc, ostrich is loaded with protein and iron.

<u>Oysters</u> – Oysters are a great source of zinc. If they're not exactly your thing, try lobster.

<u>Turkey</u> – Turkey also has the B-vitamin niacin, which specifically protects against cataracts.

<u>Wild salmon, sardines, tuna, and halibut</u> – In addition to omega-3 fats, these fish are also rich in zinc.

Other sources of zinc include: cheese, yogurt, pork, and fortified cereal.

Appendix 7
Personal care ingredients that can harm your eyes

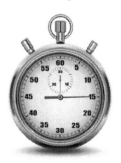

Personal care ingredients that can harm your eyes

We all introduce foreign substances to our eyes, whether on purpose or by mistake. It's often hard to figure out what it is that we are actually putting in or on us, and if we do figure it out, it's hard to know what is helpful and what is harmful.

In general, I take the view that natural products are better than synthetic products. However, this is not always the case and there is often a gray area between natural and synthetic. Most of the "good" products are natural, but there are some that have been processed to some degree or another. Some of the "bad" products are natural but still aren't very good for you. Ultimately, you need to read labels and do your own research. Also, be aware that with any ingredient, natural or otherwise, there is often some risk of an allergic reaction, so discontinue use of anything that irritates your eyes or any other part of your body.

While not exhaustive (not even close), the lists below provide some suggestions of ingredients that you might consider avoiding because they may damage your eyes or have detrimental side effects. Some ingredients are in products you put directly into your eyes (eye drops/wash and medicine), some are in products used very near the eyes (eye cream and makeup), and others are in products that can easily get in your eyes (shampoo and soap).

Since the list of things that can potentially get in your eyes is longer than can be covered here, use common sense when using personal care products that include fragrance, coloring agents, cleansing agents, etc. Be particularly careful with any spray products. Also, be aware that manufacturers use a wide variety of synonyms for ingredients, so some ingredients could be listed under another name. If you want to know about an ingredient not listed here, Appendix 8 includes some online resources for doing more in depth research.

The following list will give you a good starting point for cleaning out your medicine cabinet:

Boric acid – Found in eye drops and washes, contact lens cleaners, and saline solutions. This ingredient has been restricted in cosmetic use in Europe and Canada. It is suspected of causing reproductive toxicity.

Eyelash adhesives – Eyelash extensions are usually fixed in place by formaldehyde-based adhesives or other biologic glues. The adhesives can cause allergic reactions, as can the solvents used to remove them. In addition, cosmetic eyelash enhancers carry a risk of bacterial and fungal infection. Extensions have also been reported to cause irritation to the conjunctiva or cornea. The irritation can be caused by direct contact from the lashes themselves or hypersensitivity to the substances used to attach them.

Hydrochloric acid – Often found in eye drops, this ingredient is suspected of causing gastrointestinal or liver toxicity, immunotoxicity, asthma, skin or sense organ toxicity, and respiratory toxicity.

Imidazoline – An active ingredient in eye drops, usually listed as tetrahydrozoline, oxymetazoline, or naphazoline. Used to reduce redness in eyes, although repeated use typically makes matters worse. The FDA has issued a warning that even small amounts can be poisonous to children. While no such warning has been issued for adults, I suggest avoiding this ingredient.

Mercury – The FDA banned mercury in most cosmetics in 1974, however, they determined that mercury compounds may be used as a preservative in some eye drops and ointment. Avoid it if you can as mercury is a possible human carcinogen and human reproductive and developmental toxin.

Polypropylene – A possible carcinogen that is found in some eye shadow.

Sorbic acid – Found in many eye cosmetics, this ingredient is suspected of causing skin or sense organ toxicity. It is restricted for use in Japan.

Sulfates – These give cleansers, soaps, and shampoos their lather. Although sulfates are often derived from petroleum, they can also come from coconut and other vegetable oils that are contaminated with pesticides. Sulfates can cause eye irritation and skin rashes. They are absorbed through the skin immediately and retained in the eyes, brain, heart, and liver. Sulfates have been shown to damage eye tissue in children, delay healing of eye tissue in adults, and possibly contribute to cataract formation. The most common sulfates used in personal care products are sodium lauryl sulfate and sodium laureth sulfate.

Synthetic colors – These additives found in most eye makeup are typically made from coal tar. In addition to giving many people skin rashes, there is mounting evidence that coal tars are carcinogenic and may cause hyperactivity, ADHD, and learning difficulties in children. Coal tars can be labeled as naphtha, high solvent naphtha, naphtha distillate, benzin B70, or petroleum benzin, although artificial colors are labeled as FD&C or D&C, followed by a color and a number.

<u>Urea</u> – Usually listed as diazolidinyl urea, imidazolidinyl urea, DMDM hydantoin, or sodium hydroxymethylglycinate. This preservative, frequently found in eye makeup and eye cream, has the potential to release formaldehyde in very small amounts, is a skin irritant, and is a primary cause of contact dermatitis.

Appendix 8
Eye health resources

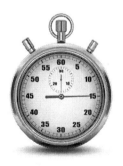

Resources

Learn more about vision and eye care:

All About Vision
www.allaboutvision.com

A comprehensive, up-to-date consumer resource about all aspects of eye health and vision correction.

The American Academy of Ophthalmology
www.geteyesmart.org

AAO's eye health information site.

The American Optometric Association
www.aoa.org

Doctor-reviewed, doctor-approved information about the most common eye conditions.

The Lighthouse National Center for Vision and Aging
www.lighthouse.org

Serves as a national clearinghouse for information on vision and aging.

Medline
www.nlm.nih.gov/medlineplus/eyesandvision.html

The National Institutes of Health's consumer information website. It has a wealth of information about diseases, conditions, and wellness issues from the National Library of Medicine .

The National Eye Institute (NEI)
www.nei.nih.gov

This branch of the National Institutes of Health (NIH) supports research on eye disease and the visual system. Their website has a wealth of information on eye conditions and eye care.

The Optometric Extension Program Foundation
www.oepf.org/

Provides excellent information on vision and the visual process.

WebMD
www.webmd.com/eye-health/

Tips for taking care of your eyes.

Research consumer product ingredients:

Environmental Working Group's Skin Deep Database
www.ewg.org/skindeep

EWG's Skin Deep Cosmetics Database is an online guide with safety ratings for more than 78,000 cosmetics and other personal care products.

GoodGuide
www.goodguide.com/

Provides information on health, environmental, and social impacts of consumer products.

Household Products Database
householdproducts.nlm.nih.gov

A comprehensive listing of the chemical ingredients, potential health effects, and manufacturers of over 6,000 widely used consumer products.

Cosmeticsinfo.org
www.cosmeticsinfo.org

Information about the safety, testing, and regulation of cosmetics and personal care products and their ingredients. Sponsored by the Personal Care Products Council, a national trade association representing the global cosmetic and personal care products industry.

U.S. Food and Drug Administration
www.fda.gov

Information on medical, cosmetic, and other personal products.

Glossary

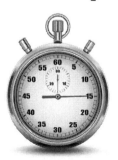

Accommodation

Eye's ability to automatically change focus from seeing at one distance to seeing at another.

Allergy

Reaction of the body's immune system to a foreign substance (e.g., pollen, animal dander, etc.). When the eyes are affected, the most common symptoms are redness, itching, tearing, swollen eyelids and stickiness.

Amblyopia

Also known as "lazy eye," amblyopia is a condition in which vision does not develop properly in one eye or the other. Amblyopia starts in childhood and, if left untreated, will prevent a child's eyes from developing correctly. As the brain matures, the eyes may not develop binocular vision and one eye will likely be weaker than the other.

Antioxidant

Substance that inhibits oxidation and can guard the body from damaging effects of free radicals (molecules with one or more unpaired electrons) which can destroy cells and play a role in many diseases. Antioxidants may help prevent macular degeneration and other eye diseases.

Astigmatism

A condition in which blurred vision is caused by the cornea being shaped more like a football than spherical like a basketball. Astigmatism may be compensated for through eyeglasses or contacts, or it can be corrected through refractive surgery.

Binocular vision

Ability of both eyes to work together to achieve proper focus, depth perception, and range of vision.

Carotenoid

A pigmented substance that adds color such as red, orange, or yellow to plants. Carotenoids have antioxidant properties.

Cataract

A condition of the crystalline lens, in which the normally clear lens becomes clouded or yellowed, causing blurred or foggy vision. Cataracts may be caused by aging, eye injuries, disease, heredity, or birth defects.

Computer vision syndrome

Collection of problems, mostly eye and vision related, associated with computer use. Symptoms include eye strain, dry eyes, blurred vision, red or pink eyes, burning, light sensitivity, headaches, and pain in the shoulders, neck and back.

Conjunctiva

The thin, normally clear, moist membrane that covers the "white" of the eye (sclera) and the inner surface of the eyelids.

Convergence

The ability to use both eyes as a team and to be able to turn the eyes inward to maintain single vision up close.

Cornea

The clear part of the eye covering the iris and pupil; it lets light into the eye, permitting sight.

Cranial nerve

One of the 12 pairs of nerves that go from the brain to other parts of the head. Those that affect the eyes and vision are the second cranial nerve (optic nerve), third (oculomotor), fourth (troclear), sixth (abducens) and seventh (facial). The optic nerve carries stimuli from the rods and cones to the brain. The third, fourth and sixth cranial nerves work with the eye muscles to control eye movement. The seventh cranial nerve works with the facial muscles to control facial movement (specifically the closure of the eyelids).

Distance vision

Generally refers to eyesight for tasks beyond arm's length, such as driving, watching television and movies, participating in sports, etc.

Double vision

Also called diplopia. When two images of the same object are perceived by one or both eyes.

Esotropia

When one or both eyes point inward, so the eyes are "crossed." This is one type of strabismus.

Exotropia

When one or both eyes point outward; also called "walleyed." This is another type of strabismus.

Glaucoma

Disease characterized by elevated intraocular pressure, which causes optic nerve damage and subsequent peripheral vision loss.

Hyperopia (farsightedness)

Condition in which the length of the eye is too short, causing light rays to focus behind the retina rather than on it, resulting in blurred near vision. Additional symptoms include eye strain and squinting.

Intermediate vision

Generally refers to eyesight at approximately arm's length, used for tasks such as computer work and viewing the speedometer in a car.

Iris

The colored membrane of the eye, surrounding the pupil. The iris controls the amount of light entering the pupil by expanding and contracting.

Irritant

A substance that consistently and predictably produces an adverse response. It can be a chemical that causes tissue inflammation at the site of contact such as reddening, swelling, itching, burning, or blistering or a physical agent causing chafing, soreness, or inflammation. Irritants are not to be confused with allergens, which induce a different cascade of reactions.

Lens

1. The nearly spherical body in the eye, located behind the cornea, that focuses light rays onto the retina.

2. A device used to focus light into the eye in order to magnify or minify images, or otherwise correct visual problems.

Macula

The most sensitive part of the retina that is about the size of a pinhead and is where our most detailed vision occurs.

Macular degeneration

Disorder characterized by changes in the eye's macula that result in the gradual loss of central vision.

Myopia (nearsightedness)

Condition in which the length of the eye is too long, causing light rays to focus in front of the retina rather than on it, resulting in blurred distance vision.

Ophthalmologist

A physician who is qualified by lengthy medical education, training, and experience to diagnose, treat, and manage all eye and visual system problems, and is licensed to practice medicine and surgery. An ophthalmologist does not typically prescribe or advocate eye exercises.

Optometrist

A health care professional who is licensed to provide primary eye care service. These services include, among other things, comprehensive eye health and vision examinations; diagnosis and treatment of eye disease and vision disorders; the prescribing of glasses, contact lenses, low vision rehabilitation, and vision therapy. The optometrist typically has an undergraduate degree and a graduate degree in optometry.

Peripheral vision

The edges of your visual field.

Presbyopia

Condition in which the aging eye beginning at around age 40 is unable to focus at all distances, often noticed when print begins to blur. Additional symptoms include eye strain, headaches, and squinting.

Pupil

The round, dark center of the eye, which opens and closes to regulate the amount of light the retina receives.

Retina

The sensory membrane that lines the back of the eye. Cells in the retina called photoreceptors transform light energy into electrical signals that are transmitted to the brain by way of the optic nerve.

Snellen chart

Standard eye chart with letters, numbers, or symbols printed in rows of decreasing size. Used by eye care professionals in distance visual acuity testing. The chart was invented by Dutch ophthalmologist Hermann Snellen.

Strabismus

A misalignment of the eyes: the eye don't point at the same object together. Crossed eyes (esotropia) are one type of strabismus; "wall-eyes" (exotropia) are another. The exact cause is unknown, but appears to be a problem with the eye muscles. Strabismus can affect depth perception.

20/20 vision

Many eye care practitioners consider this the average visual acuity for human beings, but humans can see as well as 20/15 or even 20/10. People with 20/40 vision can see clearly at 20 feet what people with 20/20 vision can see clearly at 40 feet. In most of the United States, 20/40 is the lowest uncorrected acuity required for a driver's license.

Uvea

Middle layer of the eye, below the limbus, and consisting of the iris, ciliary body, and choroid.

Visual acuity

Sharpness of vision, usually as measured with the use of a Snellen eye chart. 20/20 is considered normal visual acuity, though some people can see even better (such as 20/15 or 20/10).

Acknowledgements

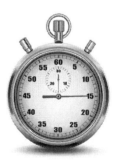

Acknowledgements

In addition to the growing challenges of age and my ongoing interest in discovering ways to better my self, my inspiration for The 15 Minute Fix came from four sources:

Tim Ferriss – The prolific author of <u>The 4-Hour Body</u> and <u>The 4-Hour Workweek</u>. Tim's desire to improve his performance in all aspects of life, his focus on quality of life, and his willingness to experiment with unconventional approaches to just about everything helped open my mind to the possibilities of what the human body may be capable of and how to stay focused on what is important in life.

Tony Horton – The outgoing creator of the P90X series of workout videos is a model for how anyone can improve their fitness level, general health, and their ability to enjoy life with minimal cost and equipment. His program is the model example of how committing to a program and making it a habitual part of your life can transform you into a new person.

Jeremy Dean – His book <u>Making Habits, Breaking Habits: Why We Do Things, Why We Don't, and How to Make Any Change Stick</u> helped me focus my thinking on how best to make The 15 Minute Fix exercise programs habitual.

My family – There is nothing I love more than being with and doing things with my family. This series ultimately evolved out of a desire to have a youthful, energetic, active life with my wife, my kids, their kids, and who knows – maybe even their kids.

The first exposure I had to the benefits of eye exercises came from Susan R. Barry's Fixing My Gaze. This is a fantastic journey of a scientist challenging scientific and medical conventional wisdom about the plasticity of the brain and possibilities of improving one's vision, even later in life. Highly recommended.

The program put forth in this book incorporates the ideas of researchers as far back as the early parts of the twentieth century up to an including work that was completed while I was writing this. The ideas of eye exercise pioneers William Bates, Frederick Brock, and A.M. Skeffington have always been considered somewhat controversial, but nevertheless provided solid starting points for thinking about eye exercises.

More recent work, such as the writings of Dr. Oliver Sacks, particularly The Mind's Eye, inspire awe and wonder at the untapped potential locked in our brains. I learned a great deal about eye concerns and training specific to athletes through Dr. Michael Peters book, See To Play. Dr. Robert Abel's writings were an excellent resource for understanding how general health (including nutrition, exercise, sleep, hydration, etc.) promotes healthy eyes, and how healthy eyes promote general health. Other recent work that I found interesting and helpful includes that of Indian researchers Dr. Nitin Gosewade, Dr. Vinod Shende, and Dr. Shriniwas Kashalikar; the research of Dr. Mitchell Scheiman; and Dr. Paul Harris's writings on behavioral optometry.

Research and educational materials out of the Mayo Clinic proved to be an invaluable resource in learning how the eyes work and how best to take care of them. I find the Mayo Clinic to be an excellent source of medical education. Their doctors and researchers are highly focused on patient needs and, as such, are open to a wide variety of approaches to care and prevention.

The 15 Minute Fix Series
So far....

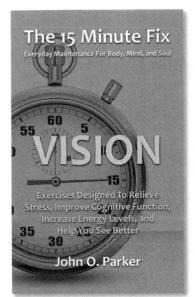

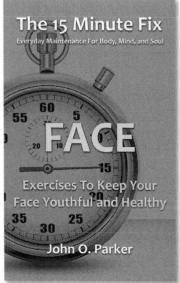

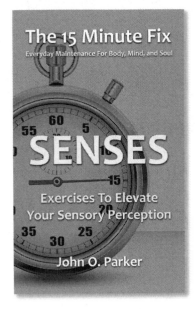

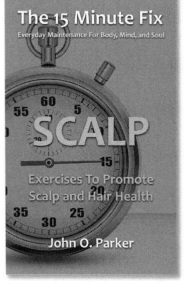

37233291R00104

Made in the USA
San Bernardino, CA
28 May 2019